FUNDAMENTALS OF
English
Grammar

FIFTH EDITION
VOLUME A

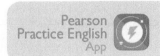

Betty S. Azar

Stacy A. Hagen

Fundamentals of English Grammar, Fifth Edition
with Pearson Practice English App
Volume A

Copyright © 2020, 2011, 2003, 1992, 1985 by Betty Schrampfer Azar
All rights reserved.

Azar Associates: Sue Van Etten, Manager

Pearson Education, 221 River Street, Hoboken, NJ 07030

Staff credits: The people who made up the *Fundamentals of English Grammar Fifth Edition* team, representing content development, design, multimedia, project management, publishing, and rights management, are Pietro Alongi, Sheila Ameri, Jennifer Castro, Tracey Cataldo, Dave Dickey, Gina DiLillo, Warren Fischbach, Sarah Henrich, Niki Lee, Stefan Machura, Amy McCormick, Robert Ruvo, Katarzyna Starzynska-Kosciuszko, Paula Van Ells, Joseph Vella, and Marcin Wozniak.

Contributing Editors: Barbara Lyons, Janice L. Baillie
Text composition: Aptara

Disclaimer: This work is produced by Pearson Education and is not endorsed by any trademark owner referenced in this publication.

Library of Congress Cataloging-in-Publication Data

A catalog record for the print edition is available from the Library of Congress.

ISBN 13: 978-0-13-511658-6
ISBN 10: 0-13-511658-9

To
Shelley Hartle and Sue Van Etten
B.S.A.

To the students and teachers at
Edmonds Community College,
from whom I learned so much
S.A.H.

Contents

Preface to the Fifth Edition

Fundamentals of English Grammar is an intermediate skills text for English language learners. It functions principally as a classroom teaching text but also serves as a comprehensive reference for students and teachers.

Using a time-tested approach that has helped millions of students around the world, *Fundamentals of English Grammar* blends direct grammar instruction with carefully sequenced practice to develop speaking, writing, listening, and reading skills. Grammar is not a mere collection of rules; rather, it is presented as a framework for organizing English. Students have a natural, logical way to help make sense of the language they see and hear.

This edition has been extensively revised to keep pace with advances in theory and practice, particularly from cognitive science. We are excited to introduce important new features and updates.

- **A pretest at the start of each chapter** allows learners to assess what they already know and orient themselves to the chapter material. Research indicates that taking a pretest may enhance learning even if a student gets every answer wrong.

- **Practice, spaced out over time**, helps students learn better. Numerous exercises have been added to provide more incremental practice.

- **New charts and exercises show patterns** to help learners make sense of the information. This reflects research showing that the adult brain is wired to look for patterns.

- **Meaning-based practice** is introduced at the sentence level. Students do not have to wait for longer passages to work with meaning, as is the case with many textbooks.

- **Frequent oral exercises** encourage students to speak more naturally and fluidly, in other words, with more automaticity—an important marker of fluency.

- **Step-by-step writing activities** promote written fluency. All end-of-chapter tasks include writing tips and editing checklists.

- **A wide range of contextualized exercises,** with an emphasis on life-skills vocabulary, encourages authentic language use.

- **Updated grammar charts** based on corpus research reflect current usage and highlight the differences between written and spoken English in formal and informal contexts.

- The **BlackBookBlog,** new to this edition, focuses on student success, cultural differences, and life-skills strategies.

- **End-of-chapter Learning Checks** help students assess their learning.

Now more than ever, teachers will find an extensive range of presentations, activities, and tasks to meet the specific needs of their classes.

Components of *Fundamentals of English Grammar,* Fifth Edition

- **Online Resources**
  - For the teacher: **Teacher's Guide** and front-of-classroom **PowerPoint** presentations
  - For the student: A Pearson Practice English **App** (with diagnostic tests, end-of-chapter Learning Checks, review tests, Student Book audio, and guided **PowerPoint** videos)
- A comprehensive **Workbook** that consists of self-study exercises for independent work
- A **Teacher's Guide** that features step-by-step teaching instructions for each chart, notes on key grammar structures, vocabulary lists, and expansion activities
- A revised **Test Bank** with quizzes, chapter tests, and mid-term and final exams
- A **Chartbook**, a reference book that consists of only the grammar charts

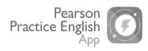

- Diagnostic tests
- End-of-chapter Learning Checks
- Review tests
- Student Book audio
- Guided PowerPoint videos

The Azar-Hagen Grammar Series consists of

- *Understanding and Using English Grammar* (blue cover), for upper-level students.
- *Fundamentals of English Grammar* (black cover), for mid-level students.
- *Basic English Grammar* (red cover), for lower or beginning levels.

Acknowledgments

We are indebted to the reviewers and other outstanding teachers who contributed to this edition by giving us extensive feedback on the Fourth edition and helping us shape the new Fifth edition.

In particular, we would like to thank Tammy Adams, University of Missouri-Kansas City; Maureen S. Andrade, Utah Valley University; Dorothy Avondstondt, Miami Dade College; Judith Campbell, University of Montreal; Shirlaine B. Castellino, Spring International Language Center, CO; Holly Cin, Houston Community College; Eileen M. Cotter, Montgomery College, MD; Yecsenia Delgado, Monrovia Adult School, CA; Andrew Donlan, International Language Institute, Washington, D.C.; Gillian L. Durham, Tidewater Community College; Jill M. Fox, University of Nebraska; Frank Grandits, City College of San Francisco; William Hennessey IV, Florida International University; Clay Hindman, Sierra Community College; Zoe Isaacson, Queens College; Barbara Jaccarino, Brooklyn College; Sharla Jones, San Antonio College; Balynda Kelly Foster, Spring International Language Center, CO; Noga Laor, Long Island University; Ann Larios, Queens College; Sara Miller, Queens College; June Ohrnberger, Suffolk County Community College, NY; Deniz Ozgorgulu, Bogazici University, Turkey; Jan Peterson, Edmonds Community College; Miriam Pollack, Grossmont College; Ray Schiel, College of English Language, Santa Monica, CA; Malek Shawareb, Houston Community College; Carol Siegel, Community College of Baltimore County; Elizabeth Marie Van Amerongen, Community College of Baltimore County; Laura Vance, Spring International Language Center, CO; Melissa Villamil, Houston Community College; Daniela C. Wagner-Loera, University of Maryland, College Park; Summer Webb, University of Colorado-Boulder; Kirsten Windahl, Cuyahoga Community College; Katarina Zorkic, Rosemead College of English.

We thank the teachers of the focus group at Edmonds Community College for their invaluable feedback: Linda Carlson, Jan Peterson, Patrick Rolland, Ruth Voetmann, and Kelly Roberts Weibel.

We once again had a stellar management and editorial team every step of the way. Product Manager Amy McCormick oversaw the project with insight and vision. We were fortunate to once again have Senior Content Producer Robert Ruvo, who deftly juggled the many components of this revision and kept us on track. Barbara Lyons, our development editor, shaped the charts, exercises, and layout with precision and care. Janice Baillie, our production editor, lent her eagle eye to every detail on every page. We are grateful as always to Sue Van Etten for her expert business management of Azar Associates.

We'd also like to thank our talented supplement writers: Geneva Tesh, Houston Community College, for the revised Workbook, MyEnglishLab, and PowerPoint material; Kelly Roberts Weibel, Edmonds Community College, for the updated Test Bank, and Ruth Voetmann, Edmonds Community College, for the reworked Teacher's Guide.

Once again, we are grateful for the Pearson design team of Tracey Cataldo and Warren Fischbach for their suggestions and expertise.

Our gratitude also goes to Pietro Alongi, Portfolio Director, and Paula Van Els, Content Development Director at Pearson. They were with the series for many years, and we appreciate the support they brought to each new edition.

Our thanks also to our illustrators Chris Pavely and Don Martinetti for their engaging artwork.

Finally, we are grateful for the support of our families as they continue to cheer us on.

Betty S. Azar
Stacy A. Hagen

Getting Started

 EXERCISE 1 ▸ Listening and reading.
Part I. Listen to the conversation between Daniel and Sofia.
They are at a college orientation. They are interviewing each other.

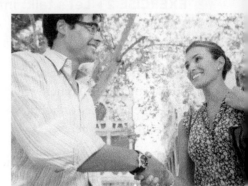

It's Nice to Meet You

DANIEL: Hi. My name is Daniel.

SOFIA: Hi. I'm Sofia. It's nice to meet you.

DANIEL: Nice to meet you too. Where are you from?

SOFIA: I'm from Montreal. How about you?

DANIEL: I'm from Miami.

SOFIA: Are you a new student?

DANIEL: Yes and no. This is my third year of college, but I'm new here.

SOFIA: This is my second year here. I'm in the business school. I really like it.

DANIEL: Oh, my major is economics! Maybe we'll have a class together. So, tell me a little more about yourself. What do you like to do in your free time?

SOFIA: I love the outdoors. I spend a lot of time in the mountains. I hike on weekends. I write about it on social media.

DANIEL: I spend a lot of time outdoors too. I like the beach. In the summer, I swim every day.

SOFIA: This town has a great beach.

DANIEL: Yeah, I want to go there! Now, when I introduce you to the group, I have to write your full name on the board. What's your last name, and how do you spell it?

SOFIA: It's Sanchez. S-A-N-C-H-E-Z.

DANIEL: My last name is Willson — with two "l"s: W-I-L-L-S-O-N.

SOFIA: Oh, it looks like our time is up. I enjoyed our conversation.

DANIEL: Thanks. I enjoyed it too.

Part II. Use the information in the conversation to complete Daniel's introduction of Sofia to the class.

DANIEL: I would like to introduce Sofia Sanchez. Sofia is from Montreal. This is her second year of college. In her free time, she...

_____

_____

_____

_____

Part III. Now it is Sofia's turn to introduce Daniel. Write her introduction. Begin with *I would like to introduce Daniel Willson*.

_____

_____

_____

_____

EXERCISE 2 ▶ Let's talk: interview.

Part I. Interview a partner.

Find out your partner's:

name (and spelling of name)
native country or hometown
free-time activities or hobbies
reason for being here

Part II. Introduce your partner to the class. After you learn each student's name, write it down.

EXERCISE 3 ▶ Writing.

Write answers to the questions. Then, with your teacher, decide what to do with your writing. See the list of suggestions at the end of the exercise.

1. What is your name?
2. Where are you from?
3. Where are you living?
4. Why are you here (in this city)?
   a. Are you a student? If so, what are you studying?
   b. Do you work? If yes, what is your job?
   c. Do you have another reason for being here?
5. What do you like to do in your free time?
6. What is your favorite season of the year? Why?
7. What are your three favorite TV programs or movies? Why do you like them?
8. Describe your first day in this class.

Suggestions for your writing:

a. Give it to a classmate to read. Your classmate can then summarize the information in a spoken report to a small group.
b. Work with a partner and correct errors in each other's writing.
c. Read your composition aloud in a small group and answer any questions about it.
d. Hand it in to your teacher, who will correct the errors and return it to you.
e. Hand it in to your teacher, who will return it at the end of the term when your English has gotten better, so you can correct your own errors.

PRETEST: What do I already know?

Choose the correct verb form in each sentence.

1. My alarm _____ at 7:00 every morning. (Chart 1-1)
   a. ring
   b. is ringing
   c. rings

2. We _____ late. (Chart 1-2)
   a. don't be
   b. aren't
   c. isn't

3. _____ right now? (Chart 1-2)
   a. Are you waiting
   b. You wait
   c. Do you wait

4. The train _____ at 5:00 every evening. (Chart 1-3)
   a. it arrives
   b. arrive
   c. arrives

5. My friend _____ several languages. (Chart 1-4)
   a. speak
   b. speakes
   c. speaks

6. _____ homework on weekends. (Chart 1-5)
   a. I have always
   b. I always have
   c. Always I have

7. I _____ the answer to your question. (Chart 1-6)
   a. am knowing
   b. know
   c. am know

8. A: Do you need more time for the test? (Chart 1-7)
   B: Yes, I _____.
   a. do
   b. am
   c. need

EXERCISE 1 ▶ Warm-up. (Charts 1-1 and 1-2)

Read the statements, and choose *yes* or *no*. Make the answers true for you. Share your answers with a partner (e.g., *I use a computer every day.* OR *I don't use a computer every day.*).

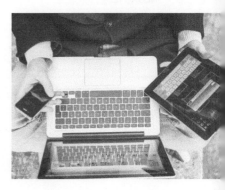

1. I use a computer or tablet every day.   yes   no

2. I am holding a tablet right now.   yes   no

3. I check emails every day.   yes   no

4. I send text messages all day long.   yes   no

5. I am sending a text message now.   yes   no

1-1 Simple Present and Present Progressive

SIMPLE PRESENT past · now · future XXXXXXXXXXXX	(a) Ann *takes* a shower *every day*. (b) I *usually read* the newspaper in the morning. (c) Babies *cry*. Birds *fly*. (d) NEGATIVE: 　It *doesn't snow* in Bangkok. (e) QUESTION: 　*Does* the teacher *speak* slowly?	The SIMPLE PRESENT expresses *daily habits* or *usual activities*, as in (a) and (b). The simple present expresses *general statements of fact,* as in (c). In general, the simple present is used for events or situations that exist always, usually, or habitually in the past, present, and future.
PRESENT PROGRESSIVE start · now · finish? in progress	(f) Ann can't come to the phone *right now* because she *is taking* a shower. (g) I *am reading* my grammar book *right now*. (h) Jimmy and Susie are babies. They *are crying right now*. Maybe they are hungry. (i) NEGATIVE: 　*It isn't snowing right now*. (j) QUESTION: 　*Is* the teacher *speaking* right now?	The PRESENT PROGRESSIVE expresses *an activity that is in progress (is occurring, is happening) right now*. The event is in progress at the time the speaker is saying the sentence. The event began in the past, is in progress now, and will probably continue into the future. FORM: ***am**, **is**, **are** + **-ing***

1-2 Forms of the Simple Present and the Present Progressive

	Simple Present				Present Progressive			
STATEMENT	I	*work.*			I	*am*	*working.*	
	You	*work.*			You	*are*	*working.*	
	He, She, It	*works.*			He, She, It	*is*	*working.*	
	We	*work.*			We	*are*	*working.*	
	They	*work.*			They	*are*	*working.*	
NEGATIVE	I	*do*	*not*	*work.*	I	*am*	*not*	*working.*
	You	*do*	*not*	*work.*	You	*are*	*not*	*working.*
	He, She, It	*does*	*not*	*work.*	He, She, It	*is*	*not*	*working.*
	We	*do*	*not*	*work.*	We	*are*	*not*	*working.*
	They	*do*	*not*	*work.*	They	*are*	*not*	*working.*
QUESTION	*Do*	I		*work?*	*Am*	I		*working?*
	Do	you		*work?*	*Are*	you		*working?*
	Does	he, she, it		*work?*	*Is*	he, she, it		*working?*
	Do	we		*work?*	*Are*	we		*working?*
	Do	they		*work?*	*Are*	they		*working?*

Contractions

pronoun + be	
	I + *am* = ***I'm*** working.
	you, we, they + *are* = ***You're, We're, They're*** working.
	he, she, it + *is* = ***He's, She's, It's*** working.

do + not			
	does + *not* = ***doesn't***	She ***doesn't*** work.
	do + *not* = ***don't***	I ***don't*** work.

be + not			
	is + *not* = ***isn't***	He ***isn't*** working.
	are + *not* = ***aren't***	They ***aren't*** working.
	(*am* + *not* = am not*	I am not working.)

*NOTE: *am* and *not* are not contracted.

EXERCISE 2 ▶ Looking at grammar. (Charts 1-1 and 1-2)

Read the paragraph. Is the activity of each verb in green a usual activity or happening right now (an activity in progress)? Write the verb in the correct column.

Lunchtime at the Café

It's noon at the café. Many students come here every day. They bring their books or laptops. They do their homework at tables. Right now some people are standing in line. A man is ordering lunch. He usually orders just coffee, but today he is hungry. Two women are talking. They are waiting to order. They meet here once a week for a study group. A man in front of them is asking questions about the food. He is taking a long time. Many people are eating at the café today. It is very busy.

USUAL ACTIVITY	RIGHT NOW
come	*are standing*

EXERCISE 3 ▸ Let's talk: pairwork. (Charts 1-1 and 1-2)

Work with a partner. Take turns completing each statement and asking a follow-up question for your partner to answer. You can look at your sentence before you speak. When you speak, look at your partner.

PARTNER A	PARTNER B
1. I usually wake up at ____ (*time*). How about you?	1. I write with my ____ (*left/right*) hand. How about you?
2. I drink ____ every morning. How about you?	2. I am living in ____ (*a dorm/an apartment/ a house, etc.*) How about you?
3. I usually eat dinner at ____ (*time*). How about you?	3. I buy a lot of ____ every week. How about you?
4. I go to bed at ____ (*time*). How about you?	4. I usually do my homework ____ (*in the morning/in the afternoon/in the evening*). How about you?
5. I'm speaking ____ (*quickly/slowly*) right now. How about you?	5. I'm looking at ____ right now. How about you?

EXERCISE 4 ▸ Reading and grammar. (Charts 1-1 and 1-2)

Choose the correct verbs.

Commuting on the Train

Lisa   takes / is taking   the train to school every day.
1

She always   meets / is meeting   her friend Ari at the station,
2

and they   sit / are sitting   together. Lisa usually
3

works / is working   on her laptop. She generally
4

does / is doing   her homework at the last minute.
5

Ari often   looks / is looking   at social media on her
6

phone and   posts / is posting   messages. Right now
7

she   doesn't post / isn't posting   anything. She
8

deletes / is deleting   photos because the memory is full.
9

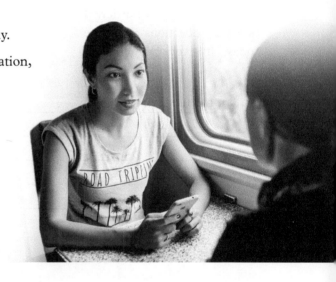

EXERCISE 5 ▸ Let's talk: pairwork. (Charts 1-1 and 1-2)

Work with a partner. Take turns describing your photos to each other and finding the differences. Use the present progressive.

PARTNER A: Cover Partner B's photos in your book.
PARTNER B: Cover Partner A's photos in your book.

Example:

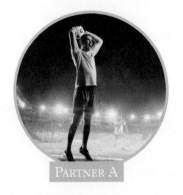

PARTNER A

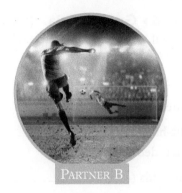

PARTNER B

PARTNER A: In my picture, a soccer player is throwing a ball.
PARTNER B: In my picture, a soccer player is kicking a ball.

PARTNER A

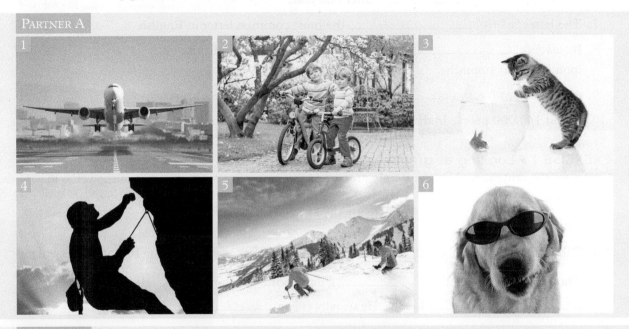

PARTNER B

EXERCISE 6 ▸ Game: trivia. (Charts 1-1 and 1-2)

Work in small groups. Complete each sentence with the correct form of the verb in parentheses. Then choose "T" for true or "F" for false. The group with the most correct answers wins.*

1. In one soccer game, a player (*run*) _____ 7 miles (11.3 km) on average.   T   F

2. In one soccer game, players (*run*) _____ 7 miles (11.3 km) on average.   T   F

3. Right-handed people (*live*) _____ 10 years longer than   T   F
   left-handed people.

4. Mountains (*cover*) _____ 3% of Africa and 25% of Europe.   T   F

5. The Eiffel Tower (*have*) _____ 3,000 steps.   T   F

6. Honey (*spoil*) _____ after one year.   T   F

7. The letter "e" (*be*) _____ the most common letter in English.   T   F

8. It (*take*) _____ about 7 seconds for food to get from our   T   F
   mouths to our stomachs.

9. A man's heart (*beat*) _____ faster than a woman's heart.   T   F

10. About 145,000 people in the world (*die*) _____ every 24 hours.   T   F

EXERCISE 7 ▸ Looking at grammar. (Charts 1-1 and 1-2)

Complete the sentences. Use the simple present or the present progressive form of the verbs in parentheses.

At Home

1. Shhh. The baby (*sleep*) __*is sleeping*__. The baby (*sleep*) __*sleeps*__ for 10 hours every night.

2. Thomas (*take*) _____ a nap on the couch right now. He (*snore*)
   _____ loudly. He usually (*snore*) _____ when he
   _____ (*sleep*).

3. Right now I'm in the kitchen. I (*sit*) _____ at the counter. I usually
   (*sit*) _____ at the counter every morning for breakfast.

4. My husband (*speak*) _____ Arabic. Arabic is his native language, but
   right now he (*speak*) _____ English on the phone to my sister.

5. A: Look outside. (*it, rain*) _____?
   B: It (*start*) _____ to sprinkle.**
   A: (*it, rain*) _____ a lot in this area?
   B: No. The weather (*be*) _____ usually warm and sunny.

---

*See *Trivia Answers*, p. 247.

**sprinkle = rain lightly

6. A: There's my neighbor Akiko. She (*leave*) _____ her house. She

(*walk*) _____ to work. Akiko (*walk*) _____ to

work every day.

B: (*you, walk*) _____ to work too?

A: Sometimes.

B: (*your husband, walk*) _____ with you?

A: No, he (*leave*) _____ for work before me.

EXERCISE 8 ▶ Let's talk. (Charts 1-1 and 1-2)
Your teacher will ask one student to perform an action and another student to describe it using the present progressive.

Example: stand next to your desk
To STUDENT A: Would you please stand next to your desk? (*Student A stands up.*)
To STUDENT B: Who is standing next to his/her desk? OR What is (Student A) doing?
  STUDENT B: (Student A) is standing next to his/her desk.

1. stand up
2. open your book
3. look at the ceiling
4. give your book to another student
5. shake your head "no"

6. hold your pen in your left hand
7. read the title of your book
8. count aloud the number of people in the classroom

EXERCISE 9 ▶ Listening. (Charts 1-1 and 1-2)
Listen to the statements about Irene and her job. Decide if the activity of each verb is a usual activity or happening right now. Choose the correct answer.

Example: You will hear: Irene works for a video game company.

  You will choose: (usual activity)   happening right now

1. usual activity   happening right now

2. usual activity   happening right now

3. usual activity   happening right now

4. usual activity   happening right now

5. usual activity   happening right now

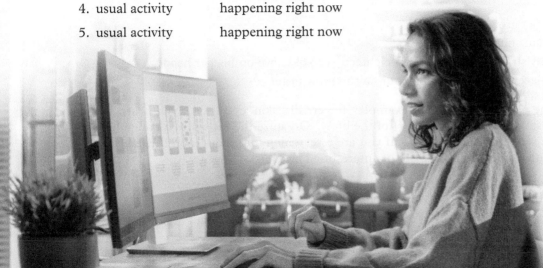

EXERCISE 10 ▶ Listening. (Charts 1-1 and 1-2)
Listen to the questions. Write the words you hear.

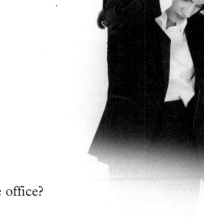

A Problem with the Printer

Example: You will hear: Is the printer working?

You will write: ___Is___ the printer working?

1. _____ need more paper?

2. _____ have enough ink?

3. _____ fixing it yourself?

4. _____ know how to fix it?

5. _____ have another printer in the office?

6. Hmmm. Is it my imagination, or _____ making a strange noise?

EXERCISE 11 ▶ Reading and writing. (Charts 1-1 and 1-2)
Part I. Read the paragraph and answer the questions.

Do you know these words?
- scalp
- strand of hair

HAIR FACTS

Here are some interesting facts about our hair. Human hair grows about one-half inch per month or 15 centimeters a year. The hair on our scalp is dead. That's why it doesn't hurt when we get a haircut. The average person has about 100,000 strands of hair. Every day we lose 75 to 150 strands of hair. One strand of hair grows for two to seven years. After it stops growing, it rests for a while and then falls out. Hair grows faster in warmer weather, and women's hair grows faster than men's hair.

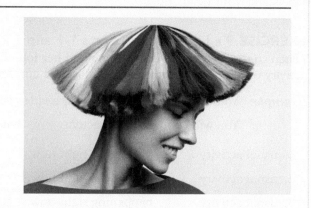

1. How fast does hair grow?
2. Why don't haircuts hurt?
3. About how many strands of hair does an eighteen-year-old have on his/her head?
4. Name a good place to live if you want your hair to grow faster.

Part II. Choose one part of the body, for example: fingernails, skin, eyebrows, eyes, heart, lungs. Make a list of interesting facts about this part of the body. Organize the facts into a paragraph. Begin with the topic sentence below. NOTE: If you are researching information on the internet, search this topic: "interesting ____ facts" (e.g., interesting hair facts).

Topic sentence: Here are some interesting facts about our ____.

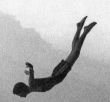

EXERCISE 12 ▶ Warm-up. (Chart 1-3)

Make sentences. Add **-s** where necessary. Do not add any other words.

1. One diver \ dive _____

2. Two diver \ dive _____

1-3 Singular / Plural

(a) SINGULAR: *one bird*	SINGULAR = one, not two or more
(b) PLURAL: *two birds, three birds, many birds, all birds, etc.*	PLURAL = two, three, or more
(c) A bird sings.	*A third person singular verb* ends in **-s**, as in (c).
(d) Birds sing.	*A plural noun* ends in **-s**, as in (d).*

(e) A *bird sings* outside my window.
  It sings loudly.
  Ann sings beautifully.
  She sings songs to her children.
  Tom sings very well.
  He sings professionally.
	A singular verb follows a singular subject.
	Add **-s** to the simple present verb if the subject is
	  (1) a singular noun (e.g., *a bird, Ann, Tom*) or
	  (2) *he, she,* or *it.***
	Note that the noun is not followed by a pronoun:
	INCORRECT: *Tom he sings very well.*

*For more information, see Chart 6-7, p. 169.

**He, *she*, and *it* are third person singular personal pronouns. See Chart 6-10, p. 175, for more information about personal pronouns.

EXERCISE 13 ▶ Looking at grammar. (Chart 1-3)

Look at each word in green. Is it a noun or verb? Is it singular or plural?

ANIMAL SOUNDS	NOUN	VERB	SING.	PLURAL
1. Cows say moo.	x			x
2. A cat meows when it's hungry.		x	x	
3. Cats meow when they are hungry.				
4. Dogs bark at squirrels.				
5. A bee buzzes in a hive.				
6. Wolves howl at night.				
7. A snake hisses when it's angry.				
8. A bat makes sounds, but people don't hear them.				

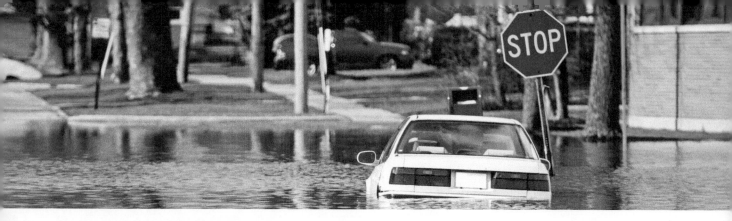

EXERCISE 14 ▸ Grammar and listening. (Chart 1-3)
Add **-s** where necessary. Write Ø if no **-s** is needed. You can check your answers by listening to the audio.

Natural Disasters: A Flood

1. The weather_Ø_ cause_s_ some natural disaster_s_.

2. Heavy rains sometimes create_____ flood_____.

3. A big flood_____ cause_____ a lot of damage.

4. In town_____, flood_____ can damage building_____, home_____, and road_____.

5. After a flood_____, a town_____ need_____ a lot of financial help for repair_____.

EXERCISE 15 ▸ Let's talk: pairwork. (Chart 1-3)
Work with a partner. One partner says the first sentence. The other completes it with a contrasting idea. Begin with *My roommate*. More than one answer may be correct. Pay attention to the third person **-s** in the completion.

Differences

1. I work in the morning.
   → *My roommate works in the evening.*
2. I exercise alone.
3. I love Italian food.
4. I drive a small car.

5. I wake up early on weekends.
6. I drink coffee every day.
7. I enjoy math.
8. I dream in English.

EXERCISE 16 ▸ Warm-up. (Chart 1-4)
Write the third person form of each verb under the correct heading. Can you figure out the rules for when to add **-s**, **-es**, and **-ies**?

drive	mix	speak	stay	study	take	try	wish

Add **-s** only.	Add **-es**.	Add **-ies**.
_____	_____	_____
_____	_____	_____
_____		
_____		

1-4 Spelling of Simple Present Verbs: Final -s/-es

(a)	visit → *visits* speak → *speaks*	Final **-s**, not **-es**, is added to most third person singular verbs. INCORRECT: *visites, speakes*
(b)	ride → *rides* write → *writes*	Many verbs end in **-e**. Final **-s** is simply added.
(c)	catch → *catches* wash → *washes* miss → *misses* fix → *fixes* buzz → *buzzes*	Final **-es** is added to verbs that end in **-ch, -sh, -s, -x,** and **-z**. PRONUNCIATION NOTE: Final **-es** is pronounced /əz/ and adds a syllable.
(d)	fly → *flies*	If a verbs ends in a consonant + **-y**, change the **-y** to **-i** and add **-es**, as in (d). INCORRECT: *flys*
(e)	pay → *pays*	If a verb ends in a vowel + **-y**, simply add **-s**,* as in (e). INCORRECT: *paies* or *payes*
(f)	go → *goes* do → *does* have → *has*	The third person singular forms of the verbs **go, do,** and ***have*** are irregular.

*Vowels = a, e, i, o, u. Consonants = all other letters in the alphabet.

EXERCISE 17 ▸ Grammar and speaking. (Chart 1-4)

Part I. Underline the verb(s) in each sentence. Add a final **-s/-es** if necessary. Do not change any other words.

What is the best way to fall asleep at night?

1. I <u>count</u> backwards from 500.

2. My wife <u>count</u>^S sheep.

3. Some people listen to white noise, like ocean waves

   or the sound of rain.

4. My doctor drinks warm milk before bedtime.

5. Yoga relax some people before they go to bed.

6. My grandmother think about a relaxing place, like

   the beach. This work well for her.

7. My best friend use a meditation technique: she breathe in and out. The in-breath take two

   seconds and the out-breath take four seconds.

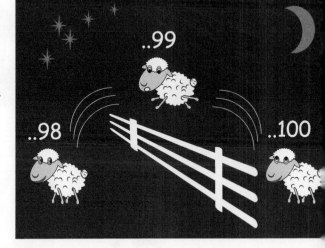

Part II. Ask three people what they do to fall asleep. Tell the class their answers.

Add *-s/-es/-ies* to the verbs. Check your answers with a partner. Listen to the pronunciation of the verbs.

1. talk_s_____
2. fish_es____
3. hope_____
4. teach_____
5. move_____

6. kiss_____
7. push_____
8. wait_____
9. mix_____
10. watch_____

11. study_____
12. buy_____
13. enjoy_____
14. try_____
15. carry_____

💬 **EXERCISE 19 ▸ Let's talk: pairwork.** (Chart 1-4)

Work with a partner. Look at the photos and make conversations. Take turns being Partner A and Partner B. Follow the model. Use *he, she,* or *they* as appropriate. You can look at the model before you speak. When you speak, look at your partner.

Example:
PARTNER A: What is he doing?
PARTNER B: He _____.
PARTNER A: Does he _____ often?
PARTNER B: Yes, he does. He _____ several times a week.

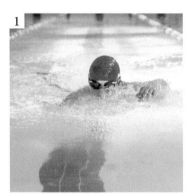

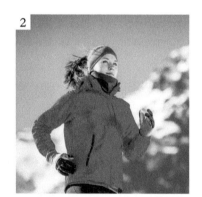

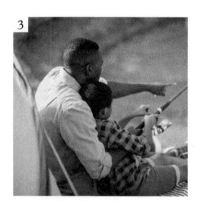

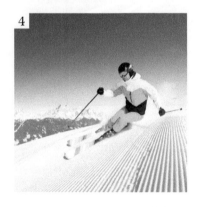

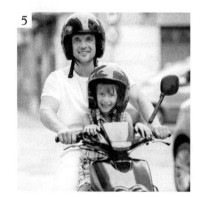

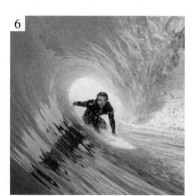

EXERCISE 20 ▸ Game. (Chart 1-4)

Work in groups of three to four students. Combine a phrase on the left with one on the right. Use each phrase once. Add **-s/-es/-ies** to the verb as necessary. Choose one person to write the sentences. The group with the most correct answers wins.

Jobs

Example: 1. A plumber
    h. fix problems with sinks and toilets
    → *A plumber fixes problems with sinks and toilets.*

1. A plumber __h__.	a. work with deposits and withdrawals of money
2. Security guards _____.	b. fix cars
3. A hospital orderly _____.	c. grow crops
4. Do bank tellers _____?	d. help doctors and nurses with nonmedical tasks
5. Auto mechanics _____.	e. cut hair, usually for men
6. An accountant _____.	f. study and prepare financial information
7. A barber _____.	g. clean buildings
8. Does a dental hygienist _____?	✓ h. fix problems with sinks and toilets
9. A janitor _____.	i. protect people and property
10. Farmers _____.	j. clean teeth

EXERCISE 21 ▸ Warm-up. (Chart 1-5)

How often do you do each activity? Give the percentage (0% → 100%). Your teacher will ask which activities you never do, sometimes do, or always do.

1. _____ I take the bus to school.

2. _____ I go to bed late.

3. _____ I skip breakfast.

4. _____ I eat vegetables at lunchtime.

5. _____ I cook my own dinner.

6. _____ I am an early riser.*

7. _____ I sleep with my phone.

8. _____ I look at social media when I wake up.

9. _____ I check the news in the middle of the night.

10. _____ I fall asleep to music.

---

early riser = a person who gets up early in the morning

1-5 Frequency Adverbs

100% ⎰ always ⎱ almost always **usually** **often** **frequently** **generally** **sometimes** **occasionally** 50% seldom rarely hardly ever almost never not ever, never 0%	Frequency adverbs usually occur in the middle of a sentence and have special positions, as shown in examples (a) through (e) below. The adverbs in **boldface** may also occur at the beginning or the end of a sentence. *I sometimes get up at 6:30.* *Sometimes I get up at 6:30.* *I get up at 6:30 sometimes.* The other adverbs in the list (not in boldface) rarely occur at the beginning or the end of a sentence. Their usual position is in the middle of a sentence.
(a) S + FREQ ADV + V Karen *always* *tells* the truth.	Except with the main verb *be,* frequency adverbs usually come between the subject and the simple present verb. INCORRECT: *Always Karen tells the truth.*
(b) S + BE + FREQ ADV Karen *is* *always* on time.	Frequency adverbs follow *be* in the simple present (*am, is, are*) and simple past (*was, were*).
(c) Do *you always eat* breakfast?	In a question, frequency adverbs come directly after the subject.
(d) Ann *usually doesn't eat* breakfast.	In a negative sentence, most frequency adverbs come in front of a negative verb (except *always* and *ever*).
(e) Sue *doesn't always eat* breakfast.	***Always*** follows a negative helping verb, as in (e), or a negative form of *be.*
(f) CORRECT: Anna *never eats* meat. INCORRECT: *Anna doesn't never eat meat.*	Negative adverbs (*seldom, rarely, hardly ever, never*) are NOT used with a negative verb.
(g) — *Do* you *ever take* the bus to work? — Yes, I do. I often take the bus.	***Ever*** is used in questions about frequency, as in (g). It means "at any time."
(h) I *don't ever walk* to work. INCORRECT: *I ever walk to work.*	***Ever*** is also used with ***not,*** as in (h). ***Ever*** is NOT used in affirmative statements.

EXERCISE 22 ▸ Grammar and speaking. (Chart 1-5)

Part I. Look at your answers in Exercise 21. Make complete sentences using the appropriate frequency word from Chart 1-5.

Examples: 1.   0% = I **never** take the bus to school.
         50% = I **often** take the bus to school.

Part II. Walk around the room and ask people about their habits.

Example: STUDENT A: I **always** take the bus to school. Do you **always** take the bus to school?
         STUDENT B: No, I don't. I **often** take the bus to school. Do you **usually** go to bed late?
         STUDENT A: Yes, I do. I **usually** go to bed late.

EXERCISE 23 ▸ Let's talk. (Chart 1-5)

Work in pairs, small groups, or as a class. Take turns asking and answering the questions. Discuss the meaning of the frequency adverbs.

What is something that ...

1. you seldom do?
2. a polite person in your country often does?
3. a polite person in your country never does?
4. our teacher frequently does in class?
5. you never do in class?
6. you rarely eat?
7. you occasionally do after class?
8. drivers generally do?
9. people in your country always or usually do to celebrate the New Year?
10. people in your country sometimes do to celebrate an important birthday?

EXERCISE 24 ▸ Looking at grammar. (Chart 1-5)

Complete the sentences using the information in the chart. Use a frequency adverb in each sentence to describe Mia's weekly activities.

MIA'S WEEK	S	M	TU	W	TH	F	S
1. wake up early				x			
2. make breakfast		x	x		x		
3. go to the gym	x	x		x		x	x
4. be late for the bus		x	x	x	x		
5. cook dinner	x	x	x	x	x	x	x
6. read a book	x	x	x	x		x	x
7. do homework			x			x	
8. go to bed early							

1. Mia _____*seldom / rarely wakes*_____ up early.

2. She _____ breakfast.

3. She _____ to the gym.

4. She _____ late for the bus.

5. She _____ dinner.

6. She _____ a book.

7. She _____ her homework.

8. She _____ to bed early.

EXERCISE 25 ▶ Let's talk: pairwork. (Charts 1-1 → 1-5)

Work with a partner. Use frequency adverbs to talk about yourself and to ask your partner questions.

Example: walk to school

PARTNER A (*book open*):   I usually walk to school. How about you? Do you usually walk to school?
PARTNER B (*book closed*): I usually walk to school too. OR
                           I seldom walk to school. I usually take the bus.

PARTNER A	PARTNER B
1. wear exercise clothes to class 2. go to sleep before 11:00 P.M. 3. check text messages during class 4. read in bed before I go to sleep 5. speak to people who sit next to me on an airplane	1. wear a hat to class 2. believe the things I hear in the news 3. get up before nine o'clock in the morning 4. call my family or a friend if I feel homesick or lonely 5. have ice cream for dessert

EXERCISE 26 ▶ Grammar and speaking. (Charts 1-1 → 1-5)

Part I. Complete the sentences with the correct simple present or present progressive form of the verbs in parentheses. Use the given frequency adverbs where necessary.

Filling out Forms

1. A: Hi, Mia. What are you doing?

   B: I (*apply*) _____ for a part-time job. I (*fill*) _____

   _____ out the application, but it (*be*) _____ difficult. I don't

   understand some of the language.

   A: I can help you.

2. You (*need, always*) _____ to use your legal name on a form.

   Your legal name (*be*) _____ on your passport or visa.

3. The phrases *last name* and *family name* (*be*) _____ the same.

4. What (*be*) _____ your middle initial?

5. For your marital status, (*be*) _____ you married, single, divorced, or widowed?

6. In the U.S., a form (*ask*) _____ for your zip code. A Canadian form (*use*) _____ the phrase *postal code*.

7. In the U.S., people (*write*) _____ "1" for the number one. In Europe, they (*do*) _____ it like this: "1". To Americans, this (*look*) _____ like the number seven. People (*write, sometimes*) _____ "7" for "7."

8. The abbreviation *DOB* (*mean*) _____ "date of birth."

9. For your DOB on U.S. forms, the month *mm* (*come, usually*) _____ first, the day *dd* (*be*) _____ second, and the year *yyyy* (*come*) _____ last.

10. Phone numbers (*have*) _____ an area code first. Some forms (*use*) _____ a hyphen, *360-555-1212*, and some forms (*use*) _____ parentheses, *(360) 555-1212*, for the area code.

Part II. With a partner, take turns finishing each sentence.

My first name is ...
My last name is ...
My middle name is ...
My middle initial is ...
My legal name is ...
My marital status is ...
My zip code/postal code is ...

EXERCISE 27 ▸ Warm-up. (Chart 1-6)
Choose the correct completions.

CHARLIE: Shhh! I _____ something on our roof.
        a. hear   b. am hearing

I _____ there is a person up there.
        a. think   b. am thinking

DAD: I _____.
        a. don't know   b. am not knowing

It _____ more like a small animal, maybe a cat or squirrel.
        a. sounds   b. is sounding

1-6 Verbs Not Usually Used in the Progressive

(a) I *know* Ms. Chen. INCORRECT: *I am knowing Ms. Chen.* (b) This book *belongs* to Mikhail. INCORRECT: *This book is belonging to Mikhail.*	Some verbs express a state or situation, not an action in progress. These verbs are called "non-action," "non-progressive," or "stative" verbs. They are generally not used in progressive tenses.*

Common Verbs That Are Generally Non-Progressive

believe	like	hear	remember	agree	own
know	need	sound	forget	disagree	belong
understand	want				
	prefer				

(c) I *think* that grammar is easy. (d) I *am thinking* about grammar right now.	Some verbs can have both progressive and non-progressive meanings. In (c): When **think** means "believe," it is non-progressive. In (d): When **think** expresses thoughts that are going through a person's mind, it can be progressive.

Common Verbs with Both Non-Progressive and Progressive Meanings

	NON-PROGRESSIVE	PROGRESSIVE
be	My grandma *is* very kind.	My grandpa *is being* difficult right now.
feel	I *feel* that you are right.	Jae *is feeling* sick today.
have	Tom *has* a car.	I *am having* a good time right now.
look	You *look* happy!	*Are* you *looking* for something?
love	Mia *loves* her husband.	Mia *is loving* retirement. She's really enjoying it.
see	*Do* you *see* the moon?	I *am seeing* my parents today.
smell	Mmmm. The soup *smells* good.	The dog *is smelling* my clothes.

*In everyday conversation, you may hear some verbs (for example, *want, like, need, hear, think*) used in the present progressive to express a state or situation: *I am wanting a sandwich. We're liking that idea.* However, the simple present is grammatically correct and more common: *I want a sandwich. We like that idea.*

EXERCISE 28 ▸ Looking at grammar. (Chart 1-6)
Choose the correct answers.

1. A: What do you like better: coffee or tea?
   B: I _____ tea.
   - a. am preferring
   - b. prefer *(circled)*

2. A: Can you help me set the table for dinner?
   B: In a minute. I _____ my report.
   - a. am finishing
   - b. finish

3. A: Are you busy?
   B: I _____ a few minutes.
   - a. am having
   - b. have

4. A: _____ a good time?
    a. Are you having   b. Do you have

   B: Yes, I _____ myself.
    a. am enjoying   b. enjoy

5. A: There goes Salma on her new racing bike.
   B: Yeah, she really _____ bikes.
    a. is loving   b. loves

   A: That's for sure! She _____ several.
    a. is owning   b. owns

EXERCISE 29 ▸ Looking at grammar. (Chart 1-6)

Complete the sentences with the simple present or present progressive form of ***think*** and ***have***.

1. A: How is your new job going?

   B: Pretty good. I (*think*) _____*think*_____ I am doing OK.

2. A: You look upset. What's on your mind?

   B: I'm worried about my daughter. I (*think*) _____ she's in trouble.

3. A: You look far away.* What's on your mind?

   B: I (*think*) _____ about my vacation next week. I can't wait!

4. A: Hey, how is the party going?

   B: Great! We (*have*) _____ fun right now.

5. A: Could I borrow some money?

   B: Sorry, I only (*have*) _____ a little change** on me.

EXERCISE 30 ▸ Looking at grammar. (Chart 1-6)

Complete the sentences. Use the simple present or present progressive form of the verbs in parentheses.

1. Right now I (*look*) _____*am looking*_____ out the window. I (*see*) _____*see*_____ a window washer on a ladder.

2. A: (*you, need*) _____ some help, Mrs. Bernini? (*you, want*)

   _____ me to carry that box for you?

   B: Yes, thank you. That's very nice of you.

3. A: Who is that man? I (*think*) _____ that I (*know*) _____

   him, but I (*forget*) _____ his name.

   B: That's Mr. Martinez.

   A: That's right! I (*remember*) _____ him now.

---

look far away = look like you are thinking about other things; daydream

**change* = coins

4. A: (*you, believe*) _____ in ghosts?

   B: No. In my opinion, ghosts (*be*) _____ only in people's imaginations.

      What (*you, think*) _____?

   A: I'm not sure. Maybe they (*be*) _____ real and maybe they (*be, not*)

      _____.

EXERCISE 31 ▶ Reading and grammar. (Charts 1-1 → 1-3, 1-6)
Choose the correct completions.

Shopping at a Clothing Store

It's Saturday at the clothing store. Many people
are shopping / shop   there today. A woman
         1
is looking / looks   at jeans. She   is seeing / sees
      2   3
several cute styles. She   is checking / checks   the sizes.
                              4
Another woman   is waiting / waits   for a dressing room.
                      5
A man   is returning / returns   a jacket at the counter.
              6
It is too big. A teenager   is checking / checks   the sales
                                  7
rack. Every week, the store   is having / has   new items
                                    8
on sale. A salesperson   is folding / folds   shirts.
                              9
Often customers   aren't folding / don't fold   them after
                        10
they   are picking / pick   them up. The salesperson
            11
is folding / folds   the clothes on the display tables several times a day.
      12
The tables   are looking / look   neat and tidy.
                  13

EXERCISE 32 ▶ Warm-up. (Chart 1-7)
Choose the correct answer for each question.

1. Does Janet eat fish?
   a. Yes, she does.   b. Yes, she is.   c. Yes, she eats.

2. Do you eat fish?
   a. No, I don't.   b. No, I am not.   c. No, I don't eat.

3. Are you vegetarian?
   a. Yes, I do.   b. Yes, I am.   c. Yes, I like.

4. Is vegetarian food popular in your country?
   a. Yes, it does.   b. Yes, it is.   c. Yes, people like.

	Question	Short Answer	Long Answer
QUESTIONS WITH *DO/DOES*	*Does* Bob *like* tea?	Yes, he *does.** No, he *doesn't.*	Yes, he likes tea.* No, he doesn't like tea.*
	Do you *like* tea?	Yes, I *do.* No, I *don't.*	Yes, I like tea. No, I don't like tea.
QUESTIONS WITH *BE*	*Are* you *studying?*	Yes, I *am.*** No, I*'m not.*	Yes, I am (I'm) studying. No, I'm not studying.
	Is Yoko a student?	Yes, she *is.** No, she*'s not.* OR No, she *isn't.*	Yes, she is (she's) a student. No, she's not a student. OR No, she isn't a student.
	Are they *studying?*	Yes, they *are.** No, they*'re not.* OR No, they *aren't.*	Yes, they are (they're) studying. No, they're not studying. OR No, they aren't studying.

*In the simple present, short answers do not include the main verb: INCORRECT: *Yes, he likes. No, he doesn't like.*

**Contractions are common in spoken English, but *am, is,* and *are* are NOT contracted with pronouns in short answers. *INCORRECT SHORT ANSWERS: Yes, I'm. Yes, she's. Yes, they're.*

EXERCISE 33 ▶ Reading and grammar. (Chart 1-7)

Part I. Read the paragraph.

Roger is 21 years old. He rides a bike every day. He lives in an area with a bicycle helmet law. The law says that helmets are necessary for everyone under 18. Roger wants to be safe. He has a new helmet, and he wears it every time he rides. Right now he is riding in the countryside. He is wearing his helmet. His brother Tom is riding his motorcycle on the highway. He is also wearing a helmet. The law requires all motorcycle riders to wear helmets.

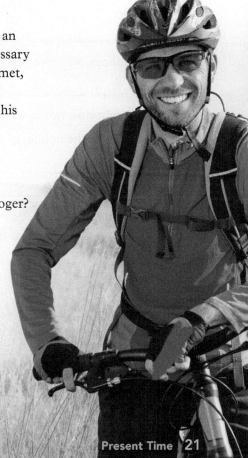

Part II. Choose the <u>expected</u> short answers.

1. Does Roger ride a bike every day?
   a. Yes, he ride.
   b. No, he doesn't.
   c. Yes, he does.
   d. No, he isn't.

2. Does his area have a bicycle helmet law?
   a. Yes, it have.
   b. Yes, it does.
   c. No, it doesn't.
   d. No, it isn't.

3. Is Tom riding with Roger?
   a. No, he isn't.
   b. No, he doesn't.
   c. Yes, he is.
   d. Yes, he does.

4. Do Roger and Tom always wear their helmets?
   a. Yes, they wear.
   b. Yes, they do.
   c. No, they aren't.
   d. No, they don't.

EXERCISE 34 ▶ Looking at grammar. (Chart 1-7)

Complete the conversations. Use the simple present or present progressive form of the verbs in parentheses. Give short answers to the questions as necessary.

Family

1. A: *(Lillian, have)* __Does Lillian have__ siblings?

   B: Yes, _____she does_____. She *(have)* _____has_____ two sisters. Lillian and her siblings

   (be) _____ triplets!

2. A: *(they, look)* _____ the same?

   B: No, _____. They *(look)* _____ different.

3. A: *(they/spend)* _____ time together during the school year?

   B: No, _____. They *(attend)* _____ different

   universities.

4. A: *(they, spend)* _____ time together right now?

   B: Yes, _____. I mean, I *(think)* _____ so

   because it's summer.

5. A: *(you, have)* _____ siblings?

   B: No, _____. I *(be)* _____ an only child. But

   I *(have)* _____ many first cousins about my age. My mom

   (come) _____ from a big family. She *(have)* _____

   11 siblings, with two sets of twins!

6. A: *(they, visit)* _____ much?

   B: Yes, right now two sisters and their kids *(stay)* _____

   with us for the holidays.

7. A: Oh, *(you, live)* _____ at home right now?

   B: Yes, _____, but I *(pay)* _____ my parents rent

   every month because now I *(work)* _____.

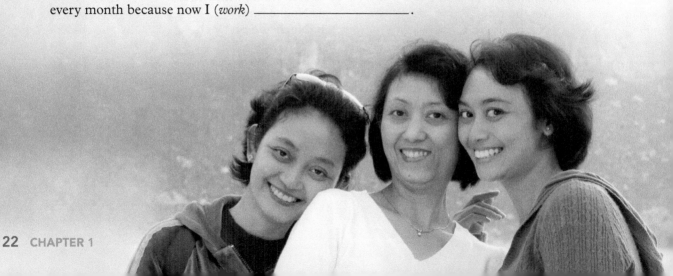

EXERCISE 35 ▸ Let's talk: pairwork. (Chart 1-7)

With a partner, complete the conversation. Practice it and then perform it for the class. You can look at your sentences before you speak. When you speak, look at your partner.

A: Do you translate from (*your language*) _____ to English when you speak?

B: (Yes/No/Sometimes) I _____.

A: Are you translating from your language right now?

B: (Yes/No) _____.

A: Do you dream in English?

B: (Yes/No/Sometimes) I _____.

A: What about you? Do you dream _____?

B: _____.

EXERCISE 36 ▸ Reading and speaking. (Chart 1-7)

Part I. Read the blog entry by co-author Stacy Hagen.

> Do you know these words?
> - strategy
> - study session

BlackBookBlog

A Technique for Remembering Information

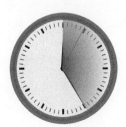

When you study, do you study for a long time and then take a break? Or do you take breaks more frequently? For many students, an hour or two seems like a good amount of time. However, studies show that your brain remembers information best at the beginning and end of your study time. The middle is actually hard to remember. If you study for an hour, you have a lot of information in the middle to remember.

Here's a strategy to help you remember more. Study for 25 minutes, and then take a 5-minute break. During this time, maybe you can check social media or get a quick snack. Then begin another 25-minute study session. When you do this, you create a new beginning, and when you finish, you create a new end. Also, the middle time is shorter, so you don't have so much information to remember. Do this a third time. If you study for 90 minutes and take these breaks, you have three beginnings and three ends. This is a better way to remember information.

Part II. Work with a partner. Answer the questions, first with a short answer and then with a long answer. Tell the class a few of your partner's answers.

1. Do you take breaks when you study?
2. Are your breaks long or short?
3. Do you look at social media during your break?

4. Is it easy for you to take just a 5-minute break? If not, why?

5. Is the technique in the blog a good technique for you? Why or why not?

 EXERCISE 37 ▶ Listening. (Chart 1-7)

Part I. Listen to these examples. Notice the reduced pronunciation of the phrases in *italics*.

At the Doctor's Office

1. Do you	→	*Dyou*	*Do you have* an appointment?
2. Does he	→	*Dze*	*Does he have* an appointment?
3. Does she	→	*Duh-she*	*Does she have* an appointment?
4. Do we	→	*Duh-we*	*Do we have* an appointment?
5. Do they	→	*Duh-they*	*Do they have* an appointment?
6. Am I	→	*Mi*	*Am I* late for my appointment?
7. Is it	→	*Zit*	*Is it* time for my appointment?★
8. Does it	→	*Zit*	*Does it* hurt?

Part II. Complete each question with the non-reduced form of the words you hear.

Example: You will hear: *Dyou* want to tell me what the problem is?

You will write: _____*Do you*_____ want to tell me what the problem is?

1. _____ have pain anywhere?

2. _____ hurt anywhere else?

3. _____ have a cough or sore throat?

4. _____ have a fever?

5. _____ need lab tests?

6. _____ very sick?

7. _____ serious?

8. _____ need to make another appointment?

9. _____ want to wait in the waiting room?

10. _____ pay now or later?

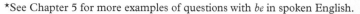

★See Chapter 5 for more examples of questions with *be* in spoken English.

EXERCISE 38 ▶ Let's talk: interview. (Chart 1-7)
Make questions. Then walk around the room and ask and answer questions. Give both a short and long answer.

Example: be \ gorillas \ intelligent?
STUDENT A: Are gorillas intelligent?
STUDENT B: Yes, they are. They are intelligent.

1. gorillas \ eat \ leaves?
2. your country \ have \ gorillas in the wild?
3. mosquitoes \ carry \ diseases?
4. the earth \ revolve \ around the sun \ right now?
5. the moon \ revolve \ around the earth \ every 28 days?

a mosquito

6. be \ the sun and moon planets?
7. be \ Toronto in western Canada?
8. be \ Texas \ in South America?
9. you \ know \ the names of the seven continents?
10. be \ our teacher \ from Australia?
11. it \ rain \ outside \ right now?
12. be \ you \ tired of this interview?

a gorilla in the wild

EXERCISE 39 ▶ Listening. (Chart 1-7)
Choose the correct answers.

Getting Ready to Leave

Example: You will hear: You're holding your keys. Are you ready to leave?
           You will choose: (a.) Yes, I am.
                             b. Yes, I do.

1. a. Yes, I want.
   b. Yes, I do.

2. a. Yes, I need.
   b. Yes, I do.

3. a. Yes, it is.
   b. Yes, it does.

4. a. Yes, we need.
   b. Yes, we do.

5. a. Yes, he does.
   b. Yes, he is.

6. a. Yes, they are.
   b. Yes, they do.

EXERCISE 40 ▶ Check your knowledge. (Chapter 1 Review)
Correct the verb errors.

Omar's Visit

1. My friend Omar ~~is owning~~ *owns* his own car now. It's brand new.*

2. Today he driving to a small town north of the city to visit his aunt.

3. He love to listen to music, so he is stream music from his phone — loudly.

4. Omar is very happy: he is drive his own car and listen to loud music.

5. Omar is visiting his aunt once a week.

6. She elderly and live alone.

7. She is thinking Omar a wonderful nephew.

8. She love his visits.

9. He try to be helpful and considerate in every way.

10. His aunt don't hearing well, so Omar is speaks loudly and clearly when he's with her.

11. When he's there, he fix things for her around her apartment and help her with her shopping.

12. He isn't staying with her overnight.

13. He usually is staying for a few hours and then is heading back to the city.

14. He kiss his aunt good-bye and give her a hug before he is leaving.

15. Omar a very good nephew.

_____

brand new = completely new

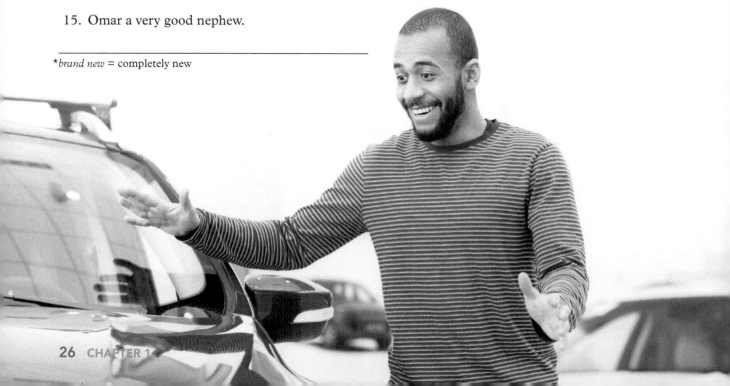

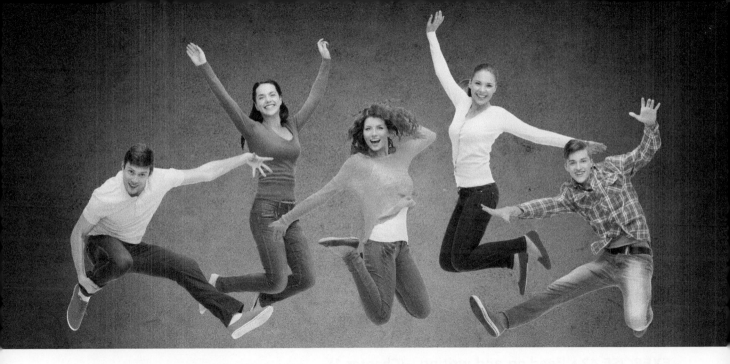

EXERCISE 41 ▶ Reading, grammar, and listening. (Chapter 1)

Part I. Read the passage.

Aerobic Exercise

Jeremy and Nancy believe exercise is important. They go to an exercise class three times a week. They like aerobic exercise.

Aerobic exercise is a special type of exercise. It increases a person's heart rate. Fast walking, running, and dancing are examples of aerobic exercise. During aerobic exercise, a person's heart beats fast. This brings more oxygen to the muscles. Muscles work longer when they have more oxygen.

Right now Jeremy and Nancy are listening to some lively music. They are doing special dance steps. They are exercising different parts of their body.

How about you? Do you like to exercise? Do your muscles get exercise every day? Do you do some type of aerobic exercise?

Do you know these words?
- oxygen
- muscles
- lively

Part II. Choose the correct verbs.

1. Jeremy and Nancy (think) / are thinking   exercise is good for them.

2. They   prefer / are preferring   aerobic exercise.

3. Aerobic exercise   makes / is making   a person's heart beat fast.

4. Muscles   need / are needing   oxygen.

5. With more oxygen, muscles   work / are working   longer.

6. Right now Jeremy and Nancy   do / are doing   a special kind of dance.

7. Do you exercise / Are you exercising   every week?

8. Do you exercise / Are you exercising   right now?

Part III. Listen to the passage and complete the sentences with the words you hear.

Many people _____ 1 aerobic exercise. It _____ 2 a special type of exercise. Aerobic exercise _____ 3 the heart beat fast. Running, fast walking, and dancing _____ 4 some examples of this exercise.

Right now some people _____ 5 in an exercise class. They _____ 6 to music, and they _____ 7. Their hearts _____ 8 fast. Many parts of their body _____ 9 exercise.

How about you? _____ 10 you exercise every day? _____ 11 you _____ 12 aerobic exercise?

EXERCISE 42 ▸ Reading and writing. (Chapter 1)

Part I. Read the paragraph. Discuss the questions that follow with a partner or in small groups.

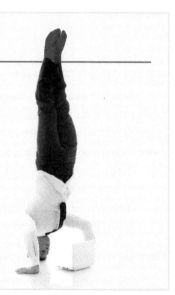

INTERESTING WAYS TO STAY FIT

Alexi doesn't have a lot of time to exercise, but he has interesting ways to stay fit. At work, he never takes the elevator. His office is on the fifth floor, and he always uses the stairs. Once a day, he walks up to the top floor of the building and then back down. When he goes home, he gets off the subway one or two stops early and walks the rest of the way home. Also, he walks very quickly. When he drives to a store, he chooses a parking space far away from the entrance. Inside the store, he balances on one leg when he waits in line to pay. He also stands on one foot when he brushes his teeth. Sometimes he watches movies at home to relax. But he doesn't relax completely. He stretches or does yoga during the movie. Alexi moves a lot during the day, and this helps keep him healthy.

1. What verb tense does the writer use? Why?
2. The main idea of the paragraph is in bold. What examples talk about interesting ways to stay fit?

Part II. Write about a healthy person you know. What does this person do to stay healthy? Does he or she exercise? Follow a special diet? Other things? Follow these steps:

1. Begin with a sentence about the person you know, and make a general statement about his/her healthy habits (main idea).
2. Give examples of the healthy habits.
3. Finish with a summary sentence: Say the main idea in different words from step 1.

WRITING TIP

When you write a paragraph, make sure to start with a topic sentence that states the main idea. Then include examples to support the topic sentence. Finish with a short summary sentence. Look at how the paragraph does this:

Topic sentence: Alexi doesn't have a lot of time to exercise, but he has interesting ways to stay fit.

Examples:
- uses stairs instead of the elevator
- walks to the top floor of the building
- gets off the subway early and walks
- walks quickly
- parks far away from the store entrance
- balances on one leg in line
- stands on one foot when he brushes his teeth
- stretches or does yoga when he watches a movie

Summary sentence: Alexi moves a lot during the day, and this helps keep him healthy.

Part III. Edit your writing. Check for the following:

1. ☐ use of the simple present to describe habits
2. ☐ correct placement of frequency adverbs
3. ☐ correct use of final *-s*/*-es*/*-ies* on singular verbs
4. ☐ topic sentence, examples, and summary sentence
5. ☐ correct spelling (use a dictionary or spell-check)

CHAPTER 1 Learning Check
Choose all the correct sentences.

1. a. My sister is owning a new car.
   b. My sister owns a new car.
   c. Do you own a car?
   d. Are you owning a car?
   e. You owning a car?

2. a. Hello! Does anyone hear me?
   b. Hello! Is anyone hearing me?
   c. Hello! Are you listening to me?
   d. Hello! Do you listen to me?

3. a. Hey, Jon. Are you downstairs?
   b. Hey, Jon. Do you downstairs?
   c. Hey, Jon. Do you here?
   d. Hey, Jon. Are you here?
   e. Hey, Jon. Are you be here?

4. a. My friend Eva a wonderful friend.
   b. My friend Eva is a wonderful friend.
   c. Always Eva has time for me.
   d. Eva always has time for me.

5. a. Irene flys for a major airline.
   b. Irene flies for a major airline.
   c. Irene is flying to Tokyo today.
   d. Irene is flieing to Tokyo today.

6. A: Do you want a snack?
   B: a. Yes, I do.
      b. Yes, I want.
      c. I no have time for a snack.
      d. I don't have time for a snack.

■■■■■ For digital resources, download the Pearson Practice English app from the Pearson English Portal (see inside front cover). Beginning with Chapter 2, all Learning Checks are available on the app.

Present Time   29

PRETEST: What do I already know?
Choose the correct answer for each sentence.

1. Our cousins _____ with us last month. (Chart 2-1)
   a. was stay   b. staying   c. stayed

2. Did you _____ last weekend? (Chart 2-1)
   a. work   b. worked   c. working

3. I _____ hungry all day yesterday. (Charts 2-2 and 2-3)
   a. felt   b. feel   c. fell

4. _____ on time for school yesterday? (Charts 2-2 and 2-3)
   a. Did you be   b. Were you   c. Are you

5. I _____ dinner last night. (Charts 2-2 and 2-3)
   a. no eat   b. didn't eat   c. didn't ate

6. My two roommates _____ last week. (Charts 2-2 and 2-3)
   a. were sick   b. sick   c. was sick

7. A car _____ suddenly in the middle of the road. (Chart 2-5)
   a. stoped   b. stopped   c. stopping

8. During the movie, the person next to me _____ the whole time. (Chart 2-6)
   a. was whispered   b. whisper   c. was whispering

9. While I _____ dinner, I heard the news about the president. (Chart 2-7)
   a. was cooking   b. cook   c. was cooked

10. _____ me a grade, my teacher read my essay. (Chart 2-8)
    a. After she gave   b. Before she gave   c. When she gave

11. Richard _____ late for class a lot, but now he comes on time. (Chart 2-9)
    a. is used to   b. used to   c. used to be

EXERCISE 1 ▸ Warm-up. (Chart 2-1)
Check (✓) the statements that are true for you. Share your answers with a partner.

1. _____ I cooked dinner last night.

2. _____ I invited my friends to join me for dinner.

3. _____ I didn't wash the dinner dishes.

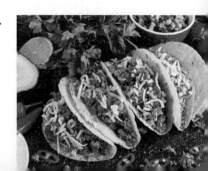

2-1 The Simple Past: Regular Verbs

(a) Mary *walked* downtown *yesterday*. (b) I *stayed* home *last weekend*.	The SIMPLE PAST is used to talk about activities or situations that began and ended in the past (e.g., *yesterday, last night, two days ago, in 2015*).
(c) Bob *played* tennis yesterday evening. (d) Our plane *landed* on time last night.	The simple past tense of most regular verbs is formed by adding *-ed* to a verb, as in (a)–(d).*

Simple Past: Regular Verb Forms

STATEMENT	NEGATIVE	QUESTION	SHORT ANSWER
I You He She } *walked*. It We They	I You He She } *did not* *walk*. It (*didn't*) We They	*Did* I *Did* you *Did* he *Did* she } *walk*? *Did* it *Did* we *Did* they	I you he Yes, she } *did*. No, it } *did not*. we (*didn't*). they

*Some verbs ending in *-y* add *-ied*, for example: *studied, worried*. See Chart 2-5. For information about pronouncing -ed endings, see Appendix A-5.

EXERCISE 2 ▸ Looking at grammar. (Chart 2-1)
Create your own chart by writing the negative and question forms of the words in *italics*.

At the Computer

	NEGATIVE	QUESTION
1. *He searched* a website.	He didn't search	Did he search
2. *They streamed* a movie.		
3. *She created* a password.		
4. *I deleted* a file.		
5. *He clicked* on a page.		
6. *She uploaded* a video.		
7. *Her computer crashed.*		
8. *It downloaded* a virus.		

EXERCISE 3 ▸ Game. (Chart 2-1)
Work with a partner or in small groups. All of the sentences contain incorrect information. Make true statements by making a negative statement and then a true statement. You can use the internet. The first team to have correct answers wins.

1. Edison invented the radio. *Edison didn't invent the radio. Edison invented the telephone.*
   OR *Edison didn't invent the radio. Marconi invented the radio.*

2. Steve Jobs started a clothing company. _____

3. Princess Diana died in a boating accident. _____

_____

4. *Apollo 1* landed on the moon. _____

_____

5. Malala Yousafzai received the Nobel Peace Prize at the age of 20. _____

_____

6. The *Titanic* crashed into a boat. _____

_____

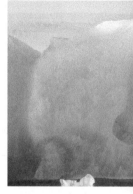

an iceberg

EXERCISE 4 ▶ Warm-up. (Charts 2-2 and 2-3)
Check (✓) the statements that are true for you.

1. _____ I slept for eight hours last night.

2. _____ I came to school on time.

3. _____ I was busy yesterday.

4. _____ I had fun last weekend.

2-2 Expressing Past Time: The Simple Past, Irregular Verbs

(a) I *ate* breakfast this morning.	Some verbs have irregular past forms, as in (a) and (b). See Chart 2-3.
(b) Sue *took* a taxi to the airport yesterday.	
(c) I *was* sick yesterday.	The simple past forms of **be** are **was** and **were**.
(d) They *were* at home last night.	

Irregular Verb Forms

STATEMENT	NEGATIVE	QUESTION	SHORT ANSWER
I You He She } *left*. It We They	I You He She } *did not* *leave*. It (*didn't*) We They	*Did* I *Did* you *Did* he *Did* she } *leave*? *Did* it *Did* we *Did* they	I you he Yes, she } *did*. No, it *did not*. we (*didn't*). they

Be Verb Forms

STATEMENT	NEGATIVE	QUESTION	SHORT ANSWER
I *was* He *was* } *nice*. She *was* It *was*	I He She } *was not* *nice*. It (*wasn't*)	*Was* I *Was* he } *nice*? *Was* she *Was* it	Yes, I, he, she, it } *was*. No, I, he, she, it } *was not*. (*wasn't*).
You *were* We *were* } *nice*. They *were*	You We } *were not* *nice*. They (*weren't*)	*Were* you *Were* we } *nice*? *Were* they	Yes, you, we, they } *were*. No, you, we, they } *were not*. (*weren't*).

2-3 Common Irregular Verbs: A Reference List

SIMPLE FORM	SIMPLE PAST	SIMPLE FORM	SIMPLE PAST	SIMPLE FORM	SIMPLE PAST
be	was, were	forgive	forgave	say	said
beat	beat	freeze	froze	see	saw
become	became	get	got	sell	sold
begin	began	give	gave	send	sent
bend	bent	go	went	set	set
bite	bit	grow	grew	shake	shook
blow	blew	hang	hung	shoot	shot
break	broke	have	had	shut	shut
bring	brought	hear	heard	sing	sang
build	built	hide	hid	sink	sank
burn	burned/burnt	hit	hit	sit	sat
buy	bought	hold	held	sleep	slept
catch	caught	hurt	hurt	slide	slid
choose	chose	keep	kept	speak	spoke
come	came	know	knew	spend	spent
cost	cost	leave	left	spread	spread
cut	cut	lend	lent	stand	stood
dig	dug	let	let	steal	stole
do	did	lie	lay	stick	stuck
draw	drew	light	lit/lighted	swim	swam
dream	dreamed/dreamt	lose	lost	take	took
drink	drank	make	made	teach	taught
drive	drove	mean	meant	tear	tore
eat	ate	meet	met	tell	told
fall	fell	pay	paid	think	thought
feed	fed	put	put	throw	threw
feel	felt	quit	quit	understand	understood
fight	fought	read	read	upset	upset
find	found	ride	rode	wake	woke/waked
fit	fit	ring	rang	wear	wore
fly	flew	rise	rose	win	won
forget	forgot	run	ran	write	wrote

EXERCISE 5 ▸ Grammar and vocabulary. (Charts 2-2 and 2-3)

Complete each sentence with the correct form of the verb in parentheses. Write the words in green under the correct photos.

At the Grocery Store

1. Daniel and Lara (*go*) _____ to the grocery store yesterday.

2. They (*walk*) _____ down the meat aisle, the produce aisle, and the dairy aisle.

3. Daniel (*push*) _____ the shopping cart.

4. Their baby (*sleep*) _____ in her car seat.

5. Lara (*hold*) _____ a shopping basket.

6. They (*see*) _____ many products on the shelves.

7. Lara (*read*) _____ the nutritional information on the packages.

8. They (*find*) _____ some good bargains.

9. Lara (*pay*) _____ the cashier at the checkout counter.

10. She (*put*) _____ the receipt in her wallet.

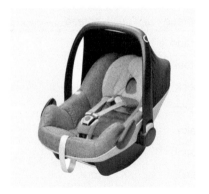

1. _____

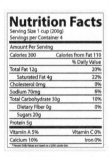

2. _____

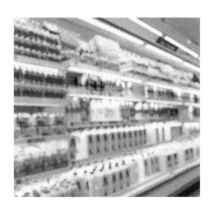

3. _____

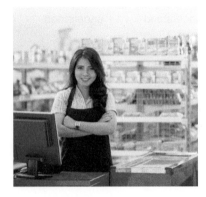

4. _____

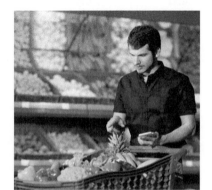

5. _____

6. _____

EXERCISE 6 ▶ Let's talk: pairwork. (Charts 2-2 and 2-3)

Make true statements for you. Write the affirmative or negative past tense form of the verb. Then tell a partner some of the things that are true for you.

1. I (*make*) <u>made / didn't make</u> a delicious dinner last night.

2. I (*speak*) _____ English with a native English speaker yesterday.

3. I (*think*) _____ about my family this morning.

4. I (*drink*) _____ coffee or tea this morning.

5. I (*ride*) _____ the bus to school today.

6. I (*send*) _____ a text message this morning.

7. I (*forget*) _____ a website password recently.

8. I (*buy*) _____ an airline ticket last year.

9. I (*swim*) _____ in a swimming pool last weekend.

10. I (*win*) _____ a sports competition when I was in school.

EXERCISE 7 ▶ Let's talk. (Charts 2-2 and 2-3)

Answer the questions. Work in pairs, small groups, or as a class.

1. What time does school begin every day? What time did your class begin today?
2. What does your teacher often tell you to do? What did he/she tell you to do today?
3. What time do you leave your home every day? What time did you leave today?
4. What do you sometimes eat for dinner? What did you eat last night?
5. What do you frequently buy at the store? What did you buy yesterday?
6. Do you get sick very often? When did you last get sick?
7. Do you take public transportation very often? When did you last take public transportation? What did it cost? How much did you pay?

EXERCISE 8 ▶ Let's talk: pairwork. (Charts 2-1 → 2-3)

Work with a partner. Ask and answer the questions with *Yes* and a complete sentence. You can look at your book before you speak. When you speak, look at your partner.

A Broken Arm

Imagine that you came to class today with a big cast on your arm. You slipped on some ice yesterday and fell down.

Example: PARTNER A: Did you have a bad day yesterday?
  PARTNER B: Yes, I had a bad day yesterday.

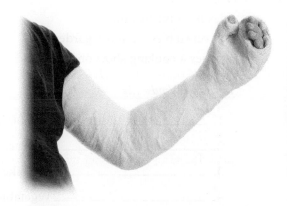

PARTNER A	PARTNER B
1. Did you fall down?	6. Did you speak with a nurse?
2. Did you hurt yourself when you fell down?	7. Did you see a doctor?
3. Did you break your arm?	8. Did the doctor put a cast on your arm?
4. Did you go to the ER (emergency room)?	9. Did you get a prescription for the pain?
5. Did you wait in the waiting room for a long time?	10. Did you pay a lot of money?

EXERCISE 9 ▶ Looking at grammar. (Charts 2-2 and 2-3)

Complete the sentences with a simple past form of a verb in the box.

bite	break	dream	eat	feel	fly	go	shake	steal

Oh, no!

1. Someone _____ my ID. Who took it?

2. I just _____ an earthquake. The house _____.

3. My sister fell on a hike and _____ her ankle.

4. We _____ on a small airplane over the mountains, and the ride was bumpy.

5. I _____ about a wolf last night. It _____ me for dinner.

6. The dog _____ our mail carrier. She _____ to an urgent care for stitches.

EXERCISE 10 ▶ Looking at grammar. (Charts 2-1 → 2-3)

Read the facts about each person. Complete the sentences with the correct form of the given verbs.

SITUATION 1: Whirlwind Wendy is energetic and does everything very quickly. Here are her typical morning activities:

wakes up at 4:00 A.M.	makes soup for dinner
cleans her apartment	brings her elderly mother a meal
rides her bike five miles	answers email messages
gets vegetables from her garden	fixes herself lunch
watches a cooking show on TV	

Yesterday, Wendy ...

1. _____woke up_____ at 4:00 A.M.

2. _____didn't clean_____ her car.

3. _____ her bike ten miles.

4. _____ vegetables from her garden.

5. _____ a comedy show on TV.

6. _____ soup for dinner.

7. _____ her elderly mother a meal.

8. _____ email messages.

9. _____ herself a snack.

SITUATION 2: Sluggish Sam doesn't get much done in a day.
Here are his typical activities:

sleeps for 12 hours	comes home
wakes up at noon	lies on the couch
takes two hours to eat breakfast	thinks about his busy life
goes fishing	begins dinner at 8:00
falls asleep on his boat	finishes dinner at 11:00

Yesterday, Sam …

1. _____*slept*_____ for 12 hours.

2. ____*didn't wake*____ up at 5:00 A.M.

3. _____ two hours to eat breakfast.

4. _____ hiking.

5. _____ asleep on his boat.

6. _____ home.

7. _____ on his bed.

8. _____ about his busy life.

9. _____ dinner at 5:00.

10. _____ dinner at 11:00.

EXERCISE 11 ▶ **Looking at grammar.** (Chart 2-3)
Complete the sentences. Use the simple past of any irregular verb that makes sense. More than one answer may be possible.

My Roommates

1. Lita walked to her job today. Rebecca _____*drove*_____ her car. Jada _____
   her bike. Yoko _____ the bus.

2. Jada had a choice between a job in finance or a job in management. She _____
   the one in management.

3. Rebecca doesn't have any money right now. She _____ it all last month.

4. Rebecca's parents _____ her a check, but she didn't get it. She's flat broke.★

5. Jada wears interesting clothes. She _____ a tuxedo to her brother's wedding last week.

6. Last night around midnight, Jada _____ some toast. She burned it, and the smoke alarm went off. It _____ everyone up.

7. Yoko's dog _____ several holes in the backyard. The grass looks terrible.

8. Lita grew up near the equator. She is enjoying the long summer days here. The sun _____ around 5:00 this morning. It _____ at 9:00 last night.

9. Lita _____ kindergarten for two years, but now she's teaching 2nd grade.

10. Yoko received a painting for her birthday. She _____ it in our living room.

EXERCISE 12 ▶ Let's talk: pairwork. (Charts 2-1 → 2-3)
With a partner, take turns asking each other to perform an action. Partner A tells Partner B to do something. Then A will ask B a question in the past tense.

Example: Open your book.
PARTNER A: Open your book.
PARTNER B: (*opens his/her book*)
PARTNER A: What did you do?
PARTNER B: I opened my book.

1. Shut your book.
2. Stand up.
3. Hide your pen.
4. Turn to page 10 in your book.
5. Put your book under your desk.
6. Write your name on a piece of paper.
Change roles.

7. Draw a bird.
8. Read a sentence from your grammar book.
9. Wave "good-bye."
10. Point to the board.
11. Spell the past tense of *speak*.
12. Repeat this question: "Which came first: the chicken or the egg?"

EXERCISE 13 ▶ Looking at grammar. (Charts 2-1 → 2-3)
Complete the conversations with the correct form of the words in parentheses.

Travel Questions

1. A: (*your plane, arrive*) *Did your plane arrive* _____ on time yesterday?

   B: Yes, *it did* _____ . It (*get*) _____ in at exactly 6:05.

2. A: (*you, sleep*) _____ on the flight?

   B: Yes, _____ . I (*sleep*) _____ for four hours.

★*flat broke* = completely out of money

3. A: (*you, take*) _____ a tour of Paris during your trip?

   B: No, _____. I (*miss*) _____ the tour because

   I (*oversleep*) _____.

   A: Why did you oversleep?

   B: I (*hear, not*) _____ my alarm.

4. A: (*you, eat*) _____ at a fancy restaurant?

   B: No, we _____. We (*have, not*) _____ enough money.

   We (*buy*) _____ food in grocery stores or small cafés.

5. A: (*you, visit*) _____ the Louvre Museum?

   B: Yes, we _____. We (*see*) _____ the *Mona Lisa*.

   A: (*Da Vinci, paint*) _____ the *Mona Lisa*?

   B: Yes, _____. He also (*paint*) _____ many other pictures.

EXERCISE 14 ▶ Let's talk: pairwork. (Charts 2-1 → 2-3)
Work with a partner. Complete the conversation. Then practice with your partner and perform it
for the class. You can look at your book before you speak. When you speak, look at your partner.

Small Talk

   A: Hi, how's it going?

   B: Good. How was your weekend?

   A: _____. I _____.

   How about you? What did you do?

   B: I _____.

   A: That sounds _____.

   B: It was.

EXERCISE 15 ▶ Let's talk: pairwork. (Charts 2-1 → 2-3)
Choose one of the company names in the box. Find out about the name on the internet. Talk to a
student who has a different company name. Follow the model. Explain vocabulary if necessary.

| Al-Jazeera® | Amazon® | CNN® | Ikea® | Samsung® |
| Alibaba® | Boeing® | Google® | LEGO® | Skype® |

Example: A: What company did you choose? (Adobe®)

   B: I chose _____*Adobe.*_____

   A: Where did the name _____*Adobe*_____ come from?

   B: ___*John Warnock was a co-founder of the company. He lived in Silicon Valley. The*___
   ___*Adobe Creek ran behind his house. Warnock named the company after the creek.*___
   ___*A creek is a small river. Here is a photo of a creek.*___

EXERCISE 16 ▸ Reading and grammar. (Charts 2-1 → 2-3)
Read the paragraph, and rewrite it in the past tense. Begin your new paragraph with **Yesterday morning**.

The Daily News

Every morning, David checks his Twitter feed. He wants to get the latest sports news. He also looks at the national news and reads several stories. His wife, Milana, checks her favorite newspapers online. She looks only at the headlines. She doesn't have a lot of time. She finishes articles later in the day. Both David and Milana know a lot about the day's events.

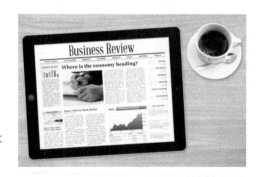

 EXERCISE 17 ▸ Warm-up: listening. (Chart 2-4)
Listen to each pair of verbs. Decide if the verb endings have the same sound or a different sound.

Example: You will hear: plays   played

You will choose: same (different)

1. same   different

2. same   different

3. same   different

4. same   different

2-4	Recognizing Verb Endings and Questions with *Did*
(a) I *agreed* with you. (b) I *agree* with you. (c) She *agrees* with you. (d) We *worked* today. (e) We *work* today. (f) He *works* today.	The **-ed** ending can be hard to hear. It can blend with the next word. For the third person simple present, you will hear an **-s** on the verb.
(g) I *was* in a hurry. (h) I *wasn't* in a hurry. (i) They *were* on time. (j) They *weren't* on time.	The "t" in an "n't" contraction can also be hard to hear. The "t" sound is not released, and you may hear just the "n."
(k) Did she → *Dih-she* (l) Did we → *Dih-we* (m) Did they → *Dih-they* (n) Did you → *Did-ja* OR *Did-ya* (o) Did I → *Dih-di* OR *Di* (p) Did he → *Dih-de* OR *De*	Note the pronunciation for questions beginning with *did*. The "d" may be dropped, as in (k)–(m). Or, the sounds may change, as in (n)–(p) At this stage of your learning, it is more important to focus on hearing the differences rather than pronouncing these words.

EXERCISE 18 ▸ Listening. (Chart 2-4)
Listen to each sentence. Choose the correct completion(s).

In the Classroom

Example: You will hear: We worked in small groups …
You will choose: a. right now   (b.) yesterday   (c.) on our project

1. a. clearly   b. every day   c. yesterday
2. a. right now   b. last week   c. to the class
3. a. almost every day   b. yesterday   c. before every test
4. a. now   b. earlier today   c. with a quiz
5. a. with native speakers b. every day   c. yesterday
6. a. in biology   b. now   c. every day
7. a. last week   b. last month   c. about fish
8. a. every week   b. last week   c. once a week

EXERCISE 19 ▸ Listening. (Chart 2-4)
Part I. Listen to the reduced pronunciations with *did*.

1. Did you   → *Did-ja*   Did you forget something?
            Did-ya   Did you forget something?
2. Did I   → *Dih-di*   Did I forget something?
            Di   Did I forget something?
3. Did he   → *Dih-de*   Did he forget something?
            De   Did he forget something?
4. Did she   → *Dih-she*   Did she forget something?
5. Did we   → *Dih-we*   Did we forget something?
6. Did they → *Dih-they* Did they forget something?

Part II. You will hear questions. Complete each answer with the pronoun and the non-reduced form of the verb you hear.

1. Yes, he _____*did*_____. He _____*cut*_____ it with a knife.

2. Yes, she _____. She _____ it all yesterday.

3. Yes, I _____. I _____ them yesterday.

4. Yes, they _____. They _____ it.

5. Yes, you _____. You _____ it.

6. Yes, she _____. She _____ them.

7. Yes, he _____ . He _____ it to him.

8. Yes, I _____ . I _____ them.

9. Yes, he _____ . He _____ it.

10. Yes, you _____ . You _____ her.

EXERCISE 20 ▶ Listening. (Chart 2-4)

Part I. The differences between **was/wasn't** and **were/weren't** can be hard to hear in spoken English. The "t" in the negative contraction is often dropped, and you may only hear an /n/ sound. Listen to these examples.

1. It was a big wedding. It wasn't a big wedding.
2. We were early. We weren't early.

Part II. Listen to these sentences about a wedding. Circle the words you hear.

At a Wedding

1. was	wasn't		6. was	wasn't
2. was	wasn't		7. was	wasn't
3. were	weren't		8. was	wasn't
4. were	weren't		9. were	weren't
5. was	wasn't		10. were	weren't

the groom and bride

EXERCISE 21 ▶ Warm-up. (Chart 2-5)

Do you know the spelling rules for these verbs?

Part I. Write the **-ing** form of each verb under the correct heading.

die   give   hit   try

Drop final **-e**. Add **-ing**.	Double final consonant. Add **-ing**.	Change **-ie** to **-y**. Add **-ing**.	Just add **-ing**.
_____	_____	_____	_____

Part II. Write the **-ed** form of each verb under the correct heading.

enjoy   tie   stop   study

Double final consonant. Add **-ed**.	Change **-y** to **-i**. Add **-ed**.	Just add **-ed**.	Just add **-d**.
_____	_____	_____	_____

2-5 Spelling of *-ing* and *-ed* Forms

End of Verb	Double the Consonant?	Simple Form	*-ing*	*-ed*	
-e	NO	(a) smile hope	smiling hoping	smiled hoped	*-ing* form: Drop the *-e*, add *-ing*. *-ed* form: Just add *-d*.
Two Consonants	NO	(b) help learn	helping learning	helped learned	If the verb ends in two consonants, just add *-ing* or *-ed*.
Two Vowels + One Consonant	NO	(c) rain heat	raining heating	rained heated	If the verb ends in two vowels + a consonant, just add *-ing* or *-ed*.
One Vowel + One Consonant	YES	**ONE-SYLLABLE VERBS**			If the verb has one syllable and ends in one vowel + one consonant, double the consonant to make the *-ing* or *-ed* form.*
		(d) stop plan	stopping planning	stopped planned	
	NO	**TWO-SYLLABLE VERBS**			If the first syllable of a two-syllable verb is stressed, do not double the consonant.
		(e) vísit óffer	visiting offering	visited offered	
	YES	(f) prefér admít	preferring admitting	preferred admitted	If the second syllable of a two-syllable verb is stressed, double the consonant.
-y	NO	(g) play enjoy	playing enjoying	played enjoyed	If the verb ends in a vowel + *-y*, keep the *-y*. Do not change the *-y* to *-i*.
		(h) worry study	worrying studying	worried studied	If the verb ends in a consonant + *-y*, keep the *-y* for the *-ing* form, but change the *-y* to *-i* to make the *-ed* form.
-ie		(i) die tie	dying tying	died tied	*-ing* form: Change the *-ie* to *-y* and add *-ing*. *-ed* form: Just add *-d*.

*EXCEPTIONS: Do not double "w" or "x": *snow, snowing, snowed, fix, fixing, fixed.*

EXERCISE 22 ▶ Looking at spelling. (Chart 2-5)
Write the *-ing* and *-ed* forms of these verbs.

	-ING	*-ED*
1. wait	_____	_____
2. clean	_____	_____
3. plant	_____	_____
4. plan	_____	_____

	-ING	**-ED**
5. hope	_____	_____
6. hop	_____	_____
7. play	_____	_____
8. study	_____	_____
9. cry	_____	_____
10. die	_____	_____
11. sleep	_____	_____ *slept (no -ed)* _____
12. run	_____	_____ *ran (no -ed)* _____

EXERCISE 23 ▶ Spelling and grammar. (Chart 2-5)

Part I. Write the correct forms.

1. begin + *ing*   _____

2. close + *ing*   _____

3. hurry + *ed*   _____

4. enjoy + *ed*   _____

5. happen + *ed*   _____

6. lie + *ing*   _____

7. listen + *ing*   _____

8. open + *ing*   _____

9. shop + *ing*   _____

10. try + *ed*   _____

Part II. Complete the sentences with the correct verb from Part I. Some are present and some are past.

At the Mall

1. We are _____ for clothes today.

2. We _____ to the mall. We wanted to be there early for the sales.

3. You look upset. What _____ ?

4. This is the wrong size. I _____ on a medium and bought a large.

5. Oh, no. The elevator door is stuck. It isn't _____ .

6. Shhh. The movie is _____ .

7. I'm _____ to an announcement. It's 9:50. The mall is

   _____ at 10:00 P.M.

8. The dressing rooms are messy. Clothes are _____ on the floor.

9. I _____ our shopping trip. It was fun.

EXERCISE 24 ▶ Reading and grammar. (Charts 2-1 → 2-5)
Complete the sentences with the correct form of the verbs in parentheses.

FROM LEMONS TO LEMONADE

There is a common saying in English: "When life gives you lemons, make lemonade." Do you understand the meaning? Lemons are sour, but lemonade is sweet. If something bad happens to you, try to make a good situation out of it.

In 2009, software engineer Brian Acton (*have*) _____

1

a bad experience. He (*need*) _____ a job. He (*apply*)

2

_____ at Twitter and Facebook. But the two famous

3

companies (*want, not*) _____ to hire him, and both (*say*)

4

_____ "no." Acton was disappointed, but he (*stay*)

5

_____ positive. He (*write*) _____ after the interview: "It (*be*)

6   7

_____ a great opportunity to connect with some fantastic people. Looking

8

forward to life's next adventure."

That same year, Acton partnered with Jan Koum, a former co-worker, and together they (*build*)

_____ WhatsApp®, a social network messaging app. Five years later, in 2014,

9

Facebook (*buy*) _____ WhatsApp for $19 billion in stock and cash. Some

10

people (*call*) _____ it a multi-billion dollar mistake, but not for Acton and

11

Koum. The company that said "no" to Acton made him an instant billionaire.

Do you know someone who made lemonade from lemons? Who? What did he or she do?

EXERCISE 25 ▶ Listening and speaking. (Charts 2-1 → 2-5)
Part I. Listen to the conversation between two friends about their weekend and answer the questions.

1. One person had a good weekend. Why?

   _____

   _____

2. His friend didn't have a good weekend. Why not?

   _____

   _____

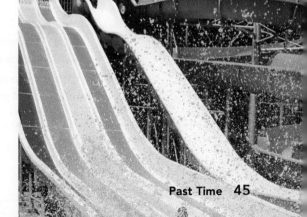

Part II. Complete the conversation with your partner. Use past tense verbs. Practice saying it until you can do it without looking at your book. Then change roles and create a new conversation. Practice it until you don't need your book. Perform one of the conversations for the class.

A: Did you have a good weekend?

B: Yeah, I _____.

A: Really? That sounds like fun!

B: It _____ great! I _____.

   How about you? How was your weekend?

A: I _____.

B: Did you have a good time?

A: Yes. / No. / Not really. _____.

EXERCISE 26 ▶ Warm-up. (Chart 2-6)
Check (✓) all the activities you were doing at midnight last night.

1. _____ I was sleeping.

2. _____ I was eating.

3. _____ I was texting.

4. _____ I was checking social media.

5. _____ I was watching a movie.

6. _____ I was having good dreams.

2-6	The Past Progressive	
PAST PROGRESSIVE 	(a) I sat down at the dinner table at 6:00 P.M. yesterday. I finished my meal at 6:30 P.M. I *was eating* dinner between 6:00 and 6:30. (b) I *was sleeping* at 9:00 last night. (c) During dinner, Sam *was checking* social media.	The PAST PROGRESSIVE expresses *an activity that was in progress (was occurring, was happening)* at a particular time in the past, as in (a)–(c). In (b), sleeping began before 9:00, was in progress at that time, and probably continued. In (c), the simple past is also correct: *During dinner, Sam checked social media.* (Meaning: He didn't continually check it.) Use of the progressive emphasizes that the activity is continuing in the past.

	(d) — Where is Jon this week?
	     — He *is traveling* on business.
	
	(e) — Jon didn't come to the party last week. I wonder why.
	     — He *was traveling* on business.
		Compare the present progressive, as in (d), with the past progressive, as in (e).

Forms of the Past Progressive			
STATEMENT		I, She, He, It	*was working.*
		You, We, They	*were working.*
NEGATIVE		I, She, He, It	*was not (wasn't) working.*
		You, We, They	*were not (weren't) working.*
QUESTION	*Was*	I, she, he, it	*working?*
	Were	you, we, they	*working?*
SHORT ANSWER	Yes,	I, she, he, it	*was.*
	No,	I, she, he, it	*wasn't.*
	Yes,	you, we, they	*were.*
	No,	you, we, they	*weren't.*

EXERCISE 27 ▸ Looking at grammar. (Chart 2-6)
Complete the sentences with a form of the verb in *italics*.

1. Our teacher *is helping* us get ready for the final exam. Yesterday at this time, he
   _____*was helping*_____ us get ready for the final exam.

2. Many students *are studying* in the library today. Yesterday, many students
   _____ in the library.

3. The registration office *is accepting* schedule changes this week. Last week the registration office
   _____ schedule changes.

4. I *am texting* my friends right now. Yesterday at this time, I _____
   my friends.

5. My roommates *are working* together on a project this afternoon. They
   _____ together yesterday afternoon too.

EXERCISE 28 ▸ Let's talk: pairwork. (Chart 2-6)
Work with a partner. Take turns asking and answering the questions. Share some of your partner's
answers with the class.

1. Were you eating breakfast at 8:00 A.M. today?
2. Were you sleeping at 11:00 P.M. yesterday?
3. What were you doing at 3:00 P.M. yesterday?
4. What were you doing between 8:00 P.M. and 9:00 P.M. last night?
5. Where were you studying six months ago?
6. Where were you living one year ago?

EXERCISE 29 ▶ Vocabulary and grammar. (Chart 2-6)

Complete the sentences with a verb in the box.

| clear off | ✓ heat up | put | rinse | set | serve | sweep |

Dinnertime

1. What were you doing at 6:00 last night?

   I _____*was heating up*_____ cold soup in the microwave.

2. What were you doing at 6:10?

   I _____ the table with spoons and napkins.

3. What were you doing at 6:15?

   I _____ dinner to my family.

4. What were you doing at 6:45?

   I _____ the table.

5. What were you doing at 6:50?

   I _____ the dishes and _____ them in the dishwasher.

6. What were you doing at 7:00?

   I _____ the floor.

EXERCISE 30 ▶ Vocabulary, reading, and grammar. (Chart 2-6)

Part I. Write the words under the correct photos.

| an outdoor faucet | a dripping faucet | a leaking pipe | a kitchen faucet |

1. _____   2. _____   3. _____   4. _____

Part II. Read the passage.

An Expensive Surprise

   The Santis had a problem. They opened their water bill and were in for an expensive surprise. Their bill was much more than usual. Instead of $100 for the month, their bill was $1,100. They checked inside their house for problems. Their bathroom sinks weren't leaking. The kitchen faucet wasn't dripping. The toilets weren't leaking. The pipes weren't broken. Then they checked outside. A water faucet was running slightly. But no one used the outdoor faucet. Then they found the answer. Their dog knew how to turn it on. The weather was unusually hot that summer. While the Santis were staying indoors with air-conditioning, he was turning on cold water to cool off. The story was funny, but the ending was not. The Santis were responsible for the entire bill. But they were glad to know they had a very smart dog.

Part III. Complete the sentences about the reading. Some verbs are negative.

1. The sinks inside the house (*cause*) _____ *weren't causing* _____ problems.

2. The bathroom sinks (*drip*) _____.

3. The toilets (*work*) _____.

4. Indoor faucets (*run*) _____.

5. The outdoor faucet (*run*) _____.

6. Their dog (*use*) _____ the faucet.

7. He (*turn*) _____ on hot water.

8. He (*cool*) _____ off with cold water.

EXERCISE 31 ▶ Looking at grammar. (Charts 1-1 and 2-6)

<u>Underline</u> the progressive verbs in the following conversations. Which are present and which are past? Discuss the way they are used. What are the similarities between the two tenses?

1. A: Where are Jan and Mark? Are they on vacation?

   B: Yes, they<u>'re traveling</u> in Kenya for a few weeks.

2. A: I invited Jan and Mark to my birthday party, but they didn't come.

   B: Why not?

   A: They were on vacation. They were traveling in Kenya.

3. A: What was I talking about when the phone interrupted me? I forget!

   B: You were describing the website you found on the internet yesterday.

4. A: I missed the beginning of the news report. What's the announcer talking about?

   B: She's describing damage from the rainstorms in Pakistan.

EXERCISE 32 ▶ Warm-up. (Chart 2-7)

<u>Underline</u> the verbs in each sentence. Which action is longer? Which one is shorter?

1. I was driving when the earthquake hit.

2. The road cracked open while I was driving.

3. While the ground was shaking, my car was moving from side to side.

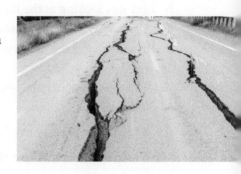

2-7 Simple Past vs. Past Progressive

SIMPLE PAST ─────╳───┼─────	(a) Maria *walked* downtown yesterday. (b) I *slept* for eight hours last night.	The simple past is used to talk about *an activity or situation that began and ended at a particular time in the past* (e.g., *yesterday, last night, two days ago, in 2014*), as in (a) and (b).
PAST PROGRESSIVE ──╳─╳─┼─────	(c) During the flight, the person next to me *was snoring* loudly.	The past progressive is used to emphasize *the duration of an activity in progress in the past.* In (c): The person was snoring from the beginning of the flight until the end.

	(d) Maria *was walking* downtown yesterday when she *saw* an old friend from high school.
	
	 (e) I *was sleeping* when a loud noise *woke* me up.
		The past progressive is used to talk about *an activity in progress (that was occurring, was happening) when another action occurred.*
		
		 In (d): First: *Maria was walking.*
		        Then: *She saw an old friend.*
		
		 In (e): First: *I was sleeping.*
		        Then: *A loud noise woke me up.*

	(f) You *were working* when I *was sleeping*. (g) While I *was doing* my homework, my roommate *was watching* a movie.	In (f) and (g): When two actions are in progress at the same time, the past progressive can be used in both parts of the sentence.
(h) *When the phone rang*, I was sleeping. (i) The phone rang *while I was sleeping*.	**when** = at that time **while** = during that time Examples (h) and (i) have the same meaning.	

EXERCISE 33 ▸ Looking at grammar. (Chart 2-7)

Read the sentences in the box and answer the questions that follow.

   a. Liza was looking at the limousine. The movie star was waving at her.
   b. Liza was looking at the limousine. The movie star waved at her.
   c. Liza looked at the limousine. The movie star was waving at her.
   d. Liza looked at the limousine. The movie star waved at her.

1. Which sentences have one longer action and one shorter action? _____ and _____

2. Which sentence has two longer actions? _____

3. Which sentence has two short actions? _____

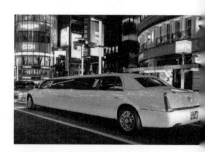

4. In Sentence b, what happened first? _____

5. In Sentence c, what happened first? _____

6. In Sentence d, what happened first? _____

EXERCISE 34 ▶ Looking at grammar. (Chart 2-7)

Complete the sentences with the simple past or past progressive form of the verbs in parentheses.

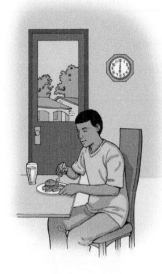 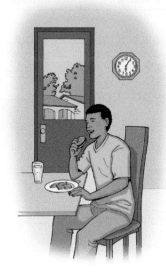 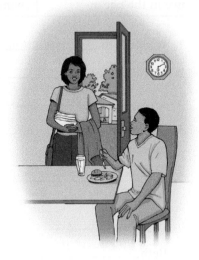

1. At 6:00 P.M. Robert sat down at the table and began to eat. At 6:05, Robert (*eat*)

   _____was eating_____ dinner.

2. While Robert (*eat*) _____ dinner, Ann (*come*) _____

   through the door.

3. In other words, when Ann (*come*) _____ through the door, Robert

   (*eat*) _____ dinner.

4. Robert went to bed at 10:30. At 11:00, Robert (*sleep*) _____ .

5. While Robert (*sleep*) _____ , his cell phone (*ring*) _____ .

6. In other words, when his cell phone (*ring*) _____ , Robert (*sleep*)

   _____ .

7. Robert left his house at 8:00 A.M. and (*begin*) _____ to walk to class.

8. While he (*walk*) _____ to class, he (*see*) _____ Mr. Ito.

9. When Robert (*see*) _____ Mr. Ito, he (*stand*) _____

   in his driveway. He (*hold*) _____ a broom.

10. Mr. Ito (*wave*) _____ once to Robert when he (*see*) _____ him.

EXERCISE 35 ▸ Looking at grammar. (Chart 2-7)

Complete the sentences, orally or in writing, using the information in the chart. Use the simple past for the shorter activity and the past progressive for the longer one.

ACTIVITY IN PROGRESS	BETH	DAVID	LILY
sit in a café	order a salad	pay a few bills	spill coffee on her lap
stand in an elevator	send a text message	run into an old friend	drop her glasses
dive in the ocean	swim past a shark	see a dolphin	find a shipwreck

1. While Beth _____*was sitting*_____ in a café, she _____*ordered*_____ a salad.

2. David _____*paid*_____ a few bills while he _____*was sitting*_____ in a café.

3. Lily _____ coffee on her lap while she _____ in a café.

4. While Beth _____ in an elevator, she _____ a text message to a friend.

5. David _____ an old friend while he _____ in an elevator.

6. Lily _____ her glasses while she _____ in an elevator.

7. Beth _____ past a shark while she _____ in the ocean.

8. While David _____ in the ocean, he _____ a dolphin.

9. While Lily _____ in the ocean, she _____ a shipwreck.

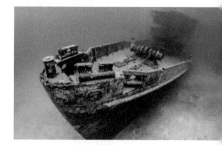

a shipwreck

EXERCISE 36 ▸ Let's talk: pairwork. (Charts 2-6 and 2-7)

Work with a partner. Take turns asking and answering the questions. You can look at your book before you speak. When you speak, look at your partner.

PARTNER A	PARTNER B
1. What were you doing at 11:00 last night?	1. What were you doing at 5:00 this morning?
2. What were you doing when the sun came up this morning?	2. What were you doing when the sun set last night?
3. What were other students doing when you walked into the classroom?	3. What were you doing when this class began?
4. What were you thinking about when you got ready for school this morning?	4. What were you thinking about when you came to school today?
5. What were you thinking when you first spoke English?	5. What were you thinking when you started this exercise?

EXERCISE 37 ▸ Reading and speaking. (Charts 2-6 and 2-7)

Your teacher will assign story A to half the class and story B to the other half of the class. Read your story several times so that you know it without looking at your book. Then tell your story to three students who have the other story. Take four minutes to tell the first person your story. Then take three minutes to tell your story to the second student. Finally, take two minutes to tell your story to the third student. The last time you speak, you should feel more comfortable than the first time.

Story A

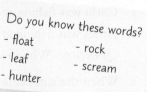

Do you know these words?
- float   - rock
- leaf   - scream
- hunter

The Ant and the Bird

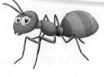

An ant was very thirsty and went to a river to drink. While he was drinking, he fell into the water. A bird was sitting in a tree and saw the ant float down the river. The ant tried to swim to safety but was unsuccessful.

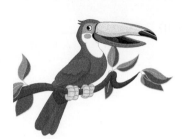

The bird flew to the ant and put a leaf close to him. The ant climbed onto the leaf and floated to the shore. While the ant was resting, a hunter came to the river. He had a rock and planned to kill the bird. The ant knew this and bit the hunter in the foot. The hunter screamed, and while he was screaming, the bird flew to safety.

Moral of the story: Kind acts lead to more kind acts.

Story B

Do you know these words?
- snore   - net
- accidentally - roar
- angrily   - escape
- hunter   - hole

The Lion and the Mouse

A mouse was running through the forest. He ran past a big lion. The lion was sleeping and snoring loudly. The mouse accidentally stepped on the lion's nose. The lion woke up and looked at the mouse angrily. "Please don't hurt me," the mouse cried. "Maybe I can help you one day." The lion laughed and put the mouse down.

A week later, a hunter's net caught the lion. The lion roared and tried to escape. While he was trying to escape, the mouse came to help him. He cut a hole in the net with his teeth. Soon the lion was free.

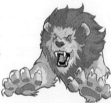

Moral of the story: Kindness brings more kindness.

EXERCISE 38 ▸ Looking at grammar. (Charts 2-6 and 2-7)
Read each pair of sentences and answer the question orally. Explain your answer.

1. a. Julia was eating breakfast. She heard the breaking news* report.
   b. Sara heard the breaking news report. She ate breakfast.
   QUESTION: Who heard the news report during breakfast? _____

2. a. Carlo was fishing at the lake. A fish was jumping out of the water.
   b. James was fishing at the lake. A fish jumped out of the water.
   QUESTION: Who saw a fish jump just one time? _____

3. a. When the sun came out, Paul walked home.
   b. When the sun came out, Vicky was walking home.
   QUESTION: Who walked home after the sun came out? _____

4. a. Joe looked at an email during class.
   b. Sam was looking at an email during class.
   QUESTION: Who probably spent more time looking at an email? _____

5. a. Pierre shouted and left the room.
   b. Olaf was shouting when he left the room.
   QUESTION: Who left after he shouted? _____

6. a. Erika was walking her dog, Hank. Hank was barking.
   b. Kate was walking her dog, Belle. Belle barked.
   QUESTION: Which dog barked more? _____

EXERCISE 39 ▸ Looking at grammar. (Chapter 1 and Charts 2-1 → 2-7)
Complete the sentences. Use the simple present, present progressive, simple past, or past progressive form of the verbs in parentheses.

Part I.

Right now Toshi and Oscar (*sit*) _____*are sitting*_____ in the library. Toshi (*do*)
                                              1
_____ his homework, but Oscar (*study, not*) _____.
            2   3
He (*stare*) _____ out the window. Toshi (*want*) _____ to know
                        4   5
what Oscar (*look*) _____ at.
                          6

TOSHI: Oscar, what (*you, look*) _____ at?
                                              7

OSCAR: I (*watch*) _____ the skateboarder. Look at that guy over there.
                          8

        He (*turn*) _____ around in circles on his back wheels. He's amazing!
                          9

---

breaking news = a special news report on the TV or radio

TOSHI: It (be) _____ 10 easier than it (look) _____ 11.

I can teach you some skateboarding basics if you'd like.

OSCAR: Great! Thanks!

Part II.

Yesterday Toshi and Oscar (sit) _____ *were sitting* _____ 12 in the library.

Toshi (do) _____ 13 his homework, but Oscar (study, not)

_____ 14. He (stare) _____ 15 out the

window. Toshi (want) _____ 16 to know what Oscar (look)

_____ 17 at. Oscar (point) _____ 18 to the skateboarder. He (say)

_____ 19 that he was amazing. Toshi (offer) _____ 20 to teach him some

skateboarding basics.

 EXERCISE 40 ▸ Grammar and listening. (Chapter 1 and Charts 2-1 → 2-7)
Choose the correct completions. You can check your answers by listening to the audio.

Jennifer's Problem

Jennifer   work / works   for an insurance company. When people   need / are needing   help
      1   2
with their car insurance, they   call / are calling   her. Right now it is 9:05 A.M., and Jennifer
                                         3
works / is working   at her desk.
        4
She   came / was coming   to work on time this morning. Yesterday Jennifer   was / is   late
           5   6
to work because she   had / was having   a car accident. While she   is driving / was driving   to
                              7   8
work, her cell phone   ring / rang. She   reached / was reaching   for it.
                              9   10
While she   is reaching / was reaching   for her phone, Jennifer   lost / was losing
                   11   12
control of the car. It   hit / was hitting   a telephone pole.
                              13
Jennifer   is / was   OK now, but her car   isn't / doesn't. She   feel / feels   very
              14   15   16
embarrassed. She   made / was making   a bad decision, especially since it is illegal
                          17
to talk on a cell phone and drive at the same time in her city.

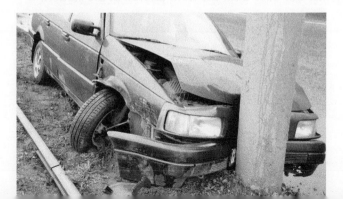

EXERCISE 41 ▶ Listening. (Charts 2-1 → 2-7)

Listen to each conversation. Then listen again and complete the sentences with the words you hear.

At a Checkout Stand in a Grocery Store

1. CASHIER: Hi. _____ what you needed?

    CUSTOMER: Almost everything. I _____ for sticky rice, but I

    _____ it.

    CASHIER: _____ on aisle 10, in the Asian food section.

2. CASHIER: This is the express lane. Ten items only. It _____ like you have more

    than ten. _____ count them?

    CUSTOMER: I _____ I _____ ten. Oh, I _____ I have

    more. Sorry.

    CASHIER: The checkout stand next to me is open.

3. CASHIER: _____ any coupons you wanted to use?

    CUSTOMER: I _____ a couple in my purse, but I can't find them now.

    CASHIER: What _____ they for? I might have some extras here.

    CUSTOMER: One _____ for eggs, and the other _____ for

    ice cream.

    CASHIER: I think I have those.

EXERCISE 42 ▶ Warm-up. (Chart 2-8)

Check (✓) the sentences that have this meaning:

First action: We gathered our bags.
Second action: The train arrived at the station.

1. _____ We gathered our bags before the train arrived at the station.

2. _____ Before the train arrived at the station, we gathered our bags.

3. _____ After we gathered our bags, the train arrived at the station.

4. _____ As soon as the train arrived at the station, we gathered our bags.

5. _____ We didn't gather our bags until the train arrived at the station.

(a) TIME CLAUSE	MAIN CLAUSE	***After I finished my work*** = a time clause*
After I finished my work,	*I went to bed.*	***I went to bed*** = a main clause

(a)

TIME CLAUSE	MAIN CLAUSE
After I finished my work,	*I went to bed.*

After I finished my work = a time clause*

I went to bed = a main clause

Examples (a) and (b) have the same meaning.

(b)

MAIN CLAUSE	TIME CLAUSE
I went to bed	*after I finished my work.*

A time clause can
   (1) come in front of a main clause, as in (a).
   (2) follow a main clause, as in (b).

(c) I went to bed *after I finished my work.*

(d) *Before I went to bed,* I finished my work.

(e) I stayed up *until I finished my work.*

(f) *As soon as I finished my work,* I went to bed.

(g) The phone rang *while I was watching* TV.

(h) *When the phone rang,* I was watching TV.

These words introduce time clauses:

> **after**
> **before**
> **until**
> **as soon as**
> **while**
> **when**

+ *subject and verb* = a time clause

In (e): *until* = to that time and then no longer**

In (f): *as soon as* = immediately after

PUNCTUATION: Put a comma at the end of a time clause when the time clause comes first in a sentence (comes in front of the main clause):

> time clause + comma + main clause
> main clause + **no** comma + time clause

(i) When the phone *rang,* I *answered* it.

In a sentence with a time clause introduced by **when**, both the time clause verb and the main verb can be simple past. In this case, the action in the **when**-clause happened first.

In (i): First: *The phone rang.*
            Then: *I answered it.*

*A clause is a structure that has a subject and a verb.

Until can also be used to say that something does NOT happen before a particular time: *I **didn't** go to bed **until** I finished my work.*

EXERCISE 43 ▶ Looking at grammar. (Chart 2-8)

Check (✓) all the clauses. Remember: A clause must have a subject and a complete verb.

   1. _____ applying for a visa

   2. _____ while the woman was applying for a visa

   3. _____ the man took passport photos

   4. _____ when the man took passport photos

   5. _____ as soon as he finished

   6. _____ he needed to finish

   7. _____ after she sent her application

   8. _____ sending her application

EXERCISE 44 ▸ Looking at grammar. (Chart 2-8)
Write "1" before the action that started first. Write "2" before the action that started second.

Taking a Taxi

1. After the taxi dropped me off, I remembered my coat in the backseat.

    a. _____ The taxi dropped me off.

    b. _____ I remembered my coat in the backseat.

2. I remembered my coat in the backseat after the taxi dropped me off.

    a. _____ I remembered my coat in the backseat.

    b. _____ The taxi dropped me off.

3. I double-checked the address before I got out of the taxi.

    a. _____ I double-checked the address.

    b. _____ I got out of the taxi.

4. Before I paid the driver, I asked for a receipt.

    a. _____ I paid the driver.

    b. _____ I asked for a receipt.

5. After I tipped the driver, he helped me with my luggage.

    a. _____ The driver helped me with my luggage.

    b. _____ I tipped the driver.

6. I tipped the driver after he helped me with my luggage.

    a. _____ I tipped the driver.

    b. _____ The driver helped me with my luggage.

EXERCISE 45 ▸ Grammar and speaking. (Chart 2-8)
Part I. Combine each set of sentences into one sentence by using a time clause. Discuss correct punctuation.

My Day

1. *First:* I cleaned up the kitchen.

    Then: I left my apartment this morning.

    Before *I left my apartment this morning, I cleaned up the kitchen.*

    I cleaned up the kitchen before *I left my apartment this morning.*

2. *First:* It began to rain.

    Then: I took out my umbrella.

    When _____

    _____ when _____

3. *First:* I worked all day.

   Then: I went home.

   After _____

   _____ after _____

4. *First:* I heard the doorbell.

   Then: I opened the door.

   As soon as _____

   _____ as soon as _____

5. *First:* I chatted with my neighbor.

   Then: I needed to go to bed.

   Until _____

   _____ until _____

6. *At the same time:* My neighbor was talking.

   I was thinking about my job.

   While _____

   _____ while _____

Part II. Work with a partner. One partner says the two sentences + the time word. The other partner, with book closed, combines the sentences. Take turns.

EXERCISE 46 ▸ Looking at grammar. (Charts 2-1 → 2-8)
Complete the sentences. Use the simple past or the past progressive form of the verbs in parentheses.

First Aid

1. I (*cut*) _____ my thumb while I (*use*)

   _____ a knife. It hurt and I

   (*yell*) _____ "Ouch." My girlfriend

   (*bring*) _____ the first-aid kit.

   bandages, tape, gauze, tablets, scissors

   She (*take*) _____ out a bandage because my thumb (*bleed*)

   _____. She (*clean*) _____ it, but the bandage (*be*)

   _____ too small, so she (*wrap*) _____ my thumb with gauze and tape.

2. A bee (*sting*) _____ Mr. Romeo on the leg when he (*plant*)

   _____ flowers. He is slightly allergic to bees. His wife (*give*)

   _____ him some medicine to help with the allergic reaction.

3. While my son (*work*) _____ at a construction site, he (*fall*)

_____ off a ladder and (*break*) _____ his ankle. He (*lie*)

_____ on the ground when some co-workers (*find*) _____

him. They (*call*) _____ 911. They (*put*) _____ ice on his ankle

and (*keep*) _____ him warm until the medics (*arrive*)_____.

EXERCISE 47 ▶ Warm-up. (Chart 2-9)

Part I. Think about your experiences when you were a beginning learner of English. Check (✓) the statements that are true for you.

When I was a beginning learner of English, ...

1. _____ I felt nervous when someone asked me a question.

2. _____ I checked my dictionary frequently.

3. _____ I asked people to speak very, very slowly.

4. _____ I translated sentences into my language a lot.

Part II. Look at the sentences you checked. Are some of these statements no longer true? If the answer is "yes," you can express your ideas with **used to**. Check (✓) the statements that are true for you.

1. _____ I used to feel nervous when someone asked me a question.

2. _____ I used to check my dictionary frequently.

3. _____ I used to ask people to speak very, very slowly.

4. _____ I used to translate sentences into my language a lot.

2-9 Expressing Past Habit: *Used To*	
(a) I *used to live* with my parents. Now I live in my own apartment.	**Used to** expresses a past situation or habit that no longer exists at present.
(b) Ann *used to be* afraid of dogs, but now she likes dogs.	FORM: **used to** + *the simple form of a verb*
(c) Al *used to smoke,* but he doesn't anymore.	
(d) *Did* you *use to live* in Paris?	QUESTION FORM: **did** + *subject* + **use to***
(e) I *didn't use to drink* coffee at breakfast, but now I always have coffee in the morning.	NEGATIVE FORM: **didn't use to**
(f) I *never used to* drink coffee at breakfast, but now I always have coffee in the morning.	*Never* can also be used to express a negative idea with *used to,* as in (f).

*Both forms **use to** and **used to** are possible in questions and negatives: **Did** *you* **used to** *live* in Paris? I **didn't used to** *drink* coffee. English language authorities do not agree on which is preferable.

EXERCISE 48 ▶ Looking at grammar. (Chart 2-9)
Make sentences with a similar meaning by using **used to**. Some of the sentences are negative, and some of them are questions.

1. When I was a child, I was shy. Now I'm not shy.

   I _____*used to be*_____ shy, but now I'm not.

2. When I was young, I thought that people over 40 were old.

   I _____ that people over 40 were old. Now I'm 40, and I don't feel old!

3. Now you live in this city. Where did you live before you came here?

   Where _____ ?

4. Did you work for the phone company at some time in the past?

   _____ for the phone company?

5. When I was younger, I slept through the night. I never woke up in the middle of the night. Now I wake up a lot.

   I _____ through the night, but now I don't.

   I _____ in the middle of the night, but now I do.

6. When I was a child, I watched cartoons on TV. I don't watch cartoons anymore. Now I stream movies.

   I _____ cartoons on TV, but I don't anymore.

   I _____ movies, but now I do.

7. How about you?

   What _____ on TV when you were little?

EXERCISE 49 ▶ Let's talk: interview. (Chart 2-9)
Walk around the classroom. Make a question with **used to** for each item. When you find a person who says "*yes*," write down his/her name and go on to the next question. Share a few of your answers with the class.

Childhood Fun

Find someone who used to …

1. play in the mud. → *Did you use to play in the mud?*
2. play with dolls or toy soldiers.
3. believe in monsters.
4. catch frogs or snakes.
5. play jokes on the teacher at school.
6. watch cartoons.
7. swing on a rope swing.

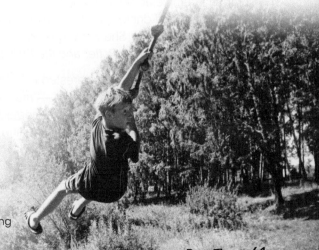

a rope swing

EXERCISE 50 ▶ Check your knowledge. (Chapter 2 Review)
Correct the errors in verb tense usage.

    1. Alex used to ~~living~~ *live* in Cairo.

    2. Did you be sick last week?

    3. Rico catched a cold after he plaied outside for several hours.

    4. My grandma lose her keys at the mall last week.

    5. Junko used to worked for an investment company.

    6. We didn't no have fun when we went to the party.

    7. Was your plane arrived on time last night?

    8. While my mom shopping, someone took her credit cards.

    9. All the students checking their phones during the class break.

   10. My family used to going to the beach every weekend, but now we don't.

EXERCISE 51 ▶ Reading and writing. (Chapter 2)
Part I. Read the passage. <u>Underline</u> the time words.

> Do you know these words?
> - journey   – take a nap
> - fame   – publisher
> - unexpected   – rejection letter
> - single mother   – wealthy

J. K. ROWLING

J. K. Rowling used to be an English language teacher before she became famous as the author of the *Harry Potter* series. From 1991 to 1994, she spent time in Portugal. While she was living there, she taught English. She was also working on her first *Harry Potter* book. Her journey from teacher to worldwide fame is an unexpected story.

After Rowling taught in Portugal, she went back to Scotland. By then she was a single mother with a young daughter. She didn't have much money, but she didn't want to return to teaching until she completed her book. Rowling did a lot of writing in a café. Her apartment was cold, and she enjoyed drinking coffee. While her daughter was taking naps beside her, Rowling worked on her book. She wrote quickly, and when her daughter was three, Rowling finished *Harry Potter and the Philosopher's Stone.**

Many publishers were not interested in her book. She doesn't remember how many rejection letters she got — maybe twelve. Finally, a small publishing company, Bloomsbury, accepted it. Shortly after its publication, the book began to sell quickly, and Rowling soon became famous. Now there are several *Harry Potter* books, and Rowling is one of the wealthiest and most successful women in the world.

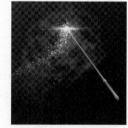

*In the United States and India, this title was changed to *Harry Potter and the Sorcerer's Stone.*

Part II. Choose a famous person you are interested in. Find information about the person's life. Make a list of important or interesting events. Then write one or more paragraphs to share this information. Use appropriate time words and expressions to help your readers follow your ideas, and edit your verbs carefully.

WRITING TIP

When you are writing about the past, it is helpful to use time words to connect some of your sentences:

Before	When	Soon	Finally
After	While	By then	Shortly after
Now			

Time words and expressions make it easier for the reader to follow your ideas. Look at what happens to the beginning of the second paragraph in the passage without time words:

> Rowling taught in Portugal. She went back to Scotland. She was a single mother with a young daughter.

It is difficult for the reader to understand exactly what happened and when. Also, the writing is "choppy" — it is not clear how the ideas connect to each other.

Part III. Edit your writing. Check for the following:

1. ☐ correct use of the simple past (a finished event)
2. ☐ correct use of the past progressive (a past event in progress)
3. ☐ use of some time words to connect ideas
4. ☐ correct spelling (use a dictionary or spell-check)

▫▫▪▪▪ For digital resources, go to the Pearson Practice English app. You can download the app from the Pearson English Portal.

PRETEST: What do I already know?

Choose the correct answers. More than one answer may be possible.

1. Thomas _____ this afternoon. (Chart 3-1)
   - a. work
   - b. will works
   - c. is going to work

2. I _____ visit my parents this evening. (Chart 3-2)
   - a. going to
   - b. am going to
   - c. am going

3. The plane will _____ at midnight. (Chart 3-3)
   - a. leave
   - b. leaves
   - c. leaving

4. It _____ all next week. (Chart 3-5)
   - a. will rain
   - b. is going to rain
   - c. rains

5. Alice _____ help us with our project. (Chart 3-6)
   - a. maybe
   - b. may be
   - c. may

6. Before you _____ work, you will need to speak with the manager. (Chart 3-7)
   - a. are leaving
   - b. will leave
   - c. leave

7. I _____ up Tom as soon as he calls. (Chart 3-7)
   - a. am going to pick
   - b. will pick
   - c. pick

8. Janelle _____ to the party tomorrow. (Chart 3-8)
   - a. comes
   - b. is going to come
   - c. is coming

9. The train _____ at 7:00 A.M. tomorrow. (Chart 3-9)
   - a. arrives
   - b. it arrives
   - c. will arrive

10. Shhh. The show _____ begin. (Chart 3-10)
    - a. about to
    - b. about
    - c. is about to

11. I am going to go to bed early and _____ in late. (Chart 3-11)
    - a. sleep
    - b. sleeping
    - c. I sleep

EXERCISE 1 ▸ Warm-up. (Chart 3-1)

Which sentences express future meaning? Do the future sentences have the same meaning or a different meaning?

1. It is going to snow today.
2. It snowed today.
3. It will snow today.

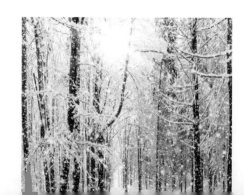

3-1 Expressing Future Time: *Be Going To* and *Will*

FUTURE	(a) I *am going to leave* at nine tomorrow morning. (b) I *will leave* at nine tomorrow morning.	*Be going to* and *will* are used to express future time. Examples (a) and (b) have the same meaning. NOTE: Sometimes *will* and *be going to* express different meanings. See Chart 3-5.
(c) Sam *is* in his office *this morning*. (d) Ann *was* in her office *this morning* at eight, but now she's at a meeting. (e) Bob *is going to be* in his office *this morning* after his dentist appointment.		*Today, tonight,* and *this* + *morning, afternoon, evening, week,* etc., can express present, past, or future time, as in (c) through (e).

NOTE: The use of *shall* (with *I* or *we*) to express future time is possible but is infrequent and quite formal; for example: *I shall* leave at nine tomorrow morning. *We shall* leave at ten tomorrow morning.

EXERCISE 2 ▸ Looking at grammar. (Chart 3-1)
Check (✓) the sentences that express future time.

At the Airport

1. _____ The security line will take about a half hour.

2. _____ The plane is going to arrive at Gate 10.

3. _____ Your flight is already an hour late.

4. _____ Your flight will be here soon.

5. _____ Did you print your boarding pass?

6. _____ Are you printing my boarding pass too?

7. _____ Are we going to have a snack on our flight?

8. _____ We will need to buy snacks on the flight.

EXERCISE 3 ▸ Looking at grammar. (Chart 3-1)
Choose all the correct completions.

At Work

1. My vacation will start	at noon.	next week.	tonight.
2. The project will be ready	this afternoon.	last night.	today.
3. Our manager is going to retire	tomorrow.	this week.	yesterday.
4. The new manager arrived	today.	this morning.	last week.
5. She spoke with us	this morning.	tonight.	today.
6. The office is going to close early	this evening.	next week.	yesterday.

EXERCISE 4 ▸ Let's talk: interview. (Chapters 1 and 2; Chart 3-1)
Make questions. Begin with the words in the box. Then walk around the room and take turns asking and answering questions. Share some of your classmates' answers with the class.

Past:	What did you do ... ?
Present:	What are you doing ... ?
	What do you do ... ?
Future:	What are you going to do ... ?

Example: yesterday → *What did you do yesterday?*

1. right now _____

2. tomorrow _____

3. every day _____

4. this month _____

5. a week from now _____

6. the day before yesterday _____

7. the day after tomorrow _____

8. last week _____

9. every week _____

10. this weekend _____

EXERCISE 5 ▸ Warm-up. (Chart 3-2)
Choose the verb in each sentence to make true statements.

1. I   am going to / am not going to   sleep in* tomorrow morning.

2. Our teacher   is going to / is not going to   retire next month.

3. We   are going to / are not going to   have a class party next week.

3-2	Forms with *Be Going To*	
(a) We *are going to be* late. (b) She*'s going to come* tomorrow. INCORRECT: *She's going to comes tomorrow.*	*Be going to* is followed by the simple form of the verb, as in (a) and (b).	

(c) *Am*   I
     Is   he, she, it ⎫ *going to be* late?
     Are   they, we, you ⎭
	QUESTION FORM: **be** + *subject* + **going to**	

(d)   I   *am not* ⎫
   He, She, It   *is not* ⎬ *going to be* late.
   They, We, You   *are not* ⎭
	NEGATIVE FORM: **be** + **not** + **going to**	

_____

*sleep in = sleep late; not wake up early in the morning

EXERCISE 6 ▶ Looking at grammar. (Charts 3-1 and 3-2)
Complete the sentences with a form of **be going to** and the words in parentheses.

Errands

1. A: Where (*Alex, go*) _____is Alex going to go_____ after work?

   B: He (*stop*) _____ at the movie theater and run some

   other errands.

   A: Why (*he, stop*) _____ at the movie theater?

   B: He left his credit card there. He (*get*) _____ it.

2. A: What (*you, do*) _____ after work?

   B: I (*pick up*) _____ a prescription at the pharmacy

   and get something for dinner.

3. A: What (*you, make*) _____ for dinner?

   B: I (*cook, not*) _____.

   I (*get*) _____ takeout.

4. A: (*you, finish*) _____ your

   errands soon?

   B: Yes, I (*finish*) _____ them in the

   next hour.

EXERCISE 7 ▶ Let's talk: pairwork. (Charts 3-1 and 3-2)
Work with a partner. Take turns asking and answering questions with **be going to**.

Examples: what \ you \ do \ after class?
PARTNER A: What are you going to do after class?
PARTNER B: I'm going to get a bite to eat* after class.

   you \ watch TV \ tonight?
PARTNER A: Are you going to watch TV tonight?
PARTNER B: Yes, I'm going to watch TV tonight. OR No, I'm not going to watch TV tonight.

1. where \ you \ go \ after your last class \ today?
2. what time \ you \ wake up \ tomorrow?
3. what \ you \ have \ for breakfast \ tomorrow?
4. you \ be \ home \ this evening?
5. where \ you \ be \ next year?
6. you \ become \ famous \ some day?
7. you \ take \ a trip \ sometime next year?
8. you \ do \ something unusual \ in the near future?

---

*get a bite to eat = get something to eat

EXERCISE 8 ▶ Let's talk: pairwork. (Chapters 1 and 2; Charts 3-1 and 3-2)
Work with a partner. Complete the conversation with your own words. Be creative! Practice your conversation and then present it to the class.

Example:
PARTNER A: I rode a skateboard to school yesterday.
PARTNER B: Really? Wow! Do you ride a skateboard to school often?
PARTNER A: Yes, I do. I ride a skateboard to school almost every day.
              Did you ride a skateboard to school yesterday?
PARTNER B: No, I didn't. I came by helicopter.
PARTNER A: Are you going to come to school by helicopter tomorrow?
PARTNER B: No, I'm not. I'm going to ride a motorcycle to school tomorrow.

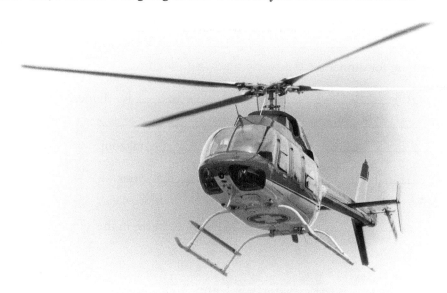

A: I _____ yesterday.

B: Really? Wow! _____ you _____ often?

A: Yes, I _____ . I _____ almost every day.

    _____ you _____ yesterday?

B: No, I _____ . I _____ .

A: Are you _____ tomorrow?

B: No, I _____ . I _____ tomorrow.

EXERCISE 9 ▶ Warm-up. (Chart 3-3)
Complete the sentences with ***will*** or ***won't***.

   1. It _____ rain tomorrow.

   2. We _____ study Chart 3-3 next.

   3. I _____ teach the class next week.

   4. *To your teacher:* You _____ need to assign homework for tonight.

3-3 Forms with *Will*

STATEMENT	I, You, She, He, It, We, They *will come* tomorrow.
NEGATIVE	I, You, She, He, It, We, They *will not (won't) come* tomorrow.
QUESTION	*Will* I, you, she, he, it, we, they *come* tomorrow?
SHORT ANSWER	Yes, No, } I, you, she, he, it, we, they { *will.** *won't.*

CONTRACTIONS	I*'ll* you*'ll*	she*'ll* he*'ll* it*'ll*	we*'ll* they*'ll*	*Will* is usually contracted with pronouns in both speech and informal writing.	

*Pronouns are NOT contracted with helping verbs in short answers.
   CORRECT: *Yes, I will.*
   INCORRECT: *Yes, I'll.*

EXERCISE 10 ▶ Looking at grammar. (Chart 3-3)
Complete the sentences with *will* and the verbs in parentheses.

Around Town

1. A new restaurant (*open*) _____ Friday night.
2. The mall (*offer*) _____ free child care tomorrow.
3. The parking garage (*close*) _____ at midnight.
4. The appliance store (*have*) _____ a sale this weekend.
5. The elementary school (*show*) _____ a family movie Friday night.
6. A band (*play*) _____ music in the park this weekend.
7. Food carts (*sell*) _____ snacks.
8. Traffic (*be*) _____ heavy in the area all weekend.

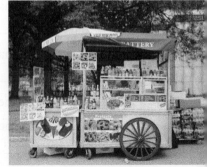

a food cart

EXERCISE 11 ▶ Let's talk: interview. (Chart 3-3)
Make complete questions with *will*. Then walk around the room and take turns asking and answering questions.

1. you \ answer my interview questions → *Will you answer my interview questions?*
2. we \ have class tomorrow?
3. it \ rain tonight?
4. the weather \ be hot next week?
5. you \ lend me some money?
6. you \ dream in English tonight?
7. we \ need our grammar books tomorrow?
8. our teacher \ give us homework today?

EXERCISE 12 ▶ Reading, grammar, and speaking. (Chart 3-3)

Part I. Read the passage.

An Old Apartment

Ted and Amy live in an old, run-down apartment and want to move.
The building has a lot of problems. The ceiling leaks when it rains. The
faucets drip. The toilet doesn't always flush properly. The windows don't
close tightly, and heat escapes from the rooms in the winter. In the
summer, it is very hot because there is no air conditioner.

Their apartment is in an unsafe part of town. Ted and Amy both take
the bus to work and need to walk a long distance to the bus stop. Their
apartment building doesn't have a laundry room, so they also have to walk
to a laundromat to wash their clothes. They are planning to have children
in the near future, so they want a park or play area nearby for their
children. A safe neighborhood is very important to them.

> Do you know these words?
> - run-down   - flush
> - ceiling   - escapes
> - leak   - air conditioner
> - faucets   - laundromat
> - drip

Part II. Ted and Amy are thinking about their next apartment and
are making a list of what they want and don't want. Complete their
sentences with **will** or **won't**.

Our Next Apartment

1. It _____ won't _____ have leaky faucets.

2. The toilet _____ flush properly.

3. It _____ have windows that close tightly.

4. There _____ be air-conditioning for hot days.

5. It _____ be in a dangerous part of town.

6. It _____ be near a bus stop.

7. There _____ be a laundry room in the building.

8. We _____ need to walk to a laundromat.

9. A play area _____ be nearby.

Part III. Imagine you are moving to a new home. Decide the six most important things you want
your home to have (*It will have ... / It won't have ...*). You can brainstorm ideas in small groups and
then discuss your ideas with the class.

EXERCISE 13 ▶ Warm-up: listening. (Chart 3-4)

Listen to the conversation. You will hear reduced speech. Choose the correct (non-reduced) form.

A: Are you _____ come with us to the meeting?   a. going   b. going to

B: No, _____ study. I have a test tomorrow.   a. I am going to   b. I am going

A: I understand. _____ you know what happens.   a. I let   b. I will let

3-4 *Be Going To* and *Will* in Spoken English

(a) You're *going to* (*gonna*) need help. (b) We're *going to* (*gonna*) be late. (c) He's *going to* (*gonna*) take the bus. (d) It's *going to* (*gonna*) rain.	In spoken English, it is common to hear *gonna* for ***going to***.
(e) I'll (*ahl*) help you. (f) You'll (*yul*) help. (g) He'll (*hill*) help you. (h) She'll (*shill*) help you. (i) We'll (*wul*) help you.	***Will*** in contractions can be difficult to hear. The vowels can change, and the contractions may sound very fast.
(j) *Dad'll* be here soon. (k) The *test'll* take an hour. (l) *Sam'll* leave before us.	In spoken English, ***will*** is often contracted with nouns, as in (j)–(l).

EXERCISE 14 ▶ Listening. (Chart 3-4)

Part I. Listen to the pronunciation of the reduced forms of ***going to*** in the conversation.

Apartment Hunting

A: We're going to look for an apartment to rent this weekend.

B: Are you going to look in this area?

A: No, we're going to search in an area closer to our jobs.

B: Is the rent going to be cheaper in that area?

A: Yes, apartment rents are definitely going to be cheaper.

B: Are you going to need to pay a deposit?

A: I'm sure we're going to need to pay the first and last month's rent.

Part II. Listen to the conversation and write the non-reduced form of the words you hear.

A: Where ___*are you going to*___ move to?
            ₁

B: We _____ look for something outside the city.
          2

   We _____ spend the weekend apartment hunting.
          3

A: What fees _____ need to pay?
                4

B: I think we _____ need to pay the first and last month's rent.
           5

A: _____ there _____ be other fees?
   6   7

B: There _____ probably _____ be an application fee and a cleaning
        8   9

   fee. Also, the landlord _____ probably _____ check our credit, so we
                10   11

   _____ need to pay for that.
      12

Complete the sentences with the words you hear.

Before the Party

1. We'll need to get the house ready for the party tomorrow, but _____ be gone in the morning.

2. _____ need to fold the laundry and dust the furniture.

3. I talked to your sister. _____ clean the kitchen.

4. Your dad will be home. _____ vacuum the carpets.

5. Your brothers won't be home. _____ do the cleanup.

6. Some of the guests are going to come early. _____ need to be ready by 5:00.

🎧 **EXERCISE 16 ▶ Listening.** (Chart 3-4)

Part I. Listen to the sentences. Notice the pronunciation of the contractions with nouns.

At the Doctor's Office

1. The doctor'll be with you in a few minutes.
2. Your appointment'll take about an hour.
3. Your fever'll be gone in a few days.
4. Your stitches'll disappear over the next two weeks.
5. The nurse'll schedule your tests.
6. The lab'll have the results next week.
7. The receptionist at the front desk'll set up* your next appointment.

Part II. Listen to the sentences and write the words you hear. Write the full form of the contractions.

At the Pharmacy

1. Your prescription _____*will be*_____ ready in ten minutes.

2. The medicine _____ you feel a little tired.

3. The pharmacist _____ your doctor's office.

4. This cough syrup _____ your cough.

5. Two aspirin _____ enough.

6. The generic** drug _____ less.

7. This information _____ all the side effects*** for this medicine.

---

set up = schedule

**generic* = medicine with no brand name

***side effects* = reactions, often negative, that a patient can have from a medicine

EXERCISE 17 ▸ Warm-up. (Chart 3-5)

In which conversation does Speaker B have a prior plan (a plan made before the moment of speaking)?

1. A: Oh, are you leaving?
   B: Yes. I'm going to pick up my kids at school. They have dentist appointments.

2. A: Excuse me, Mrs. Jones. The nurse from your son's school is on the phone. She said he has a fever and needs to go home.
   B: OK. Please tell her I'll be there in 20 minutes.

3-5	*Be Going To* vs. *Will*	
(a)	She *is going to succeed* because she works hard.	*Be going to* and *will* mean the same when they are used to make predictions about the future.
(b)	She *will succeed* because she works hard.	Examples (a) and (b) have the same meaning.
(c)	I bought some wood because I *am going to build* a bookcase for my apartment.	*Be going to* (but not *will*) is used to express a prior plan (i.e., a plan made before the moment of speaking). In (c): The speaker plans to build a bookcase.
(d)	This chair is too heavy for you to carry alone. I'*ll help* you.	*Will* (but not *be going to*) is used to express a decision the speaker makes at the moment of speaking. In (d): The speaker decides or volunteers to help at the immediate present moment; he did not have a prior plan or intention to help.

EXERCISE 18 ▸ Looking at grammar. (Chart 3-5)

Look at the verbs in green. Is the speaker expressing plans made before the moment of speaking (prior plans)? If so, circle *yes*. If not, circle *no*.

PRIOR PLAN?

1. A: Did you return Carmen's phone call?
   B: No, I forgot. Thanks for reminding me. I'll call her right away.   yes   no

2. A: I'm going to call Martha later this evening. Do you want to talk to her too?
   B: No, I don't think so.   yes   no

3. A: Jakob is in town for a few days.
   B: Really? Great! I'll give him a call. Is he staying at his Aunt Lara's?   yes   no

4. A: Alex is in town for a few days.
   B: I know. He called me yesterday. We're going to get together for dinner after I get off work tonight.   yes   no

5. A: I need some fresh air. I'm going for a short walk.
   B: I'll come with you.   yes   no

6. A: I'm going to take Hamid to the airport tomorrow morning.
   Do you want to come along?   yes   no
   B: Sure.

7. A: We're going to go to Uncle Scott's over the break.   yes   no
   Are you interested in coming with us?
   B: I'm not sure. I'll think about it. When do you need to know?   yes   no

EXERCISE 19 ▸ Looking at grammar. (Chart 3-5)
Restate the sentences. Use **be going to** because they are prior plans.

My Trip to Thailand

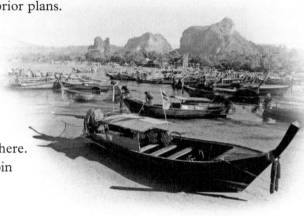

1. I'm planning to be away for three weeks.
   → *I'm going to be away for three weeks.*
2. My husband and I are planning to stay in small
   towns and camp on the beach.
3. We're planning to bring a tent.
4. We're planning to celebrate our wedding anniversary there.
5. My father, who was born in Thailand, is planning to join
   us, but he's planning to stay in a hotel.
6. He's planning to show us his favorite sights.

EXERCISE 20 ▸ Looking at grammar. (Chart 3-5)
Complete the sentences with **be going to** or **will**. Use **be going to** to express a prior plan.

1. A: Are you going by the post office today? I need to mail this letter.

   B: Yeah, I _'ll____ mail it for you.

   A: Thanks.

2. A: Why are you carrying that package?

   B: It's for my sister. I _'m going to_____ mail it to her.

3. A: Why did you buy so many eggs?

   B: I _____ make a special dessert.

4. A: I have a book for Joe from Rachel. I'm not going to see him today.

   B: Let me have it. I _____ give it to him. He's in my algebra class.

5. A: Did you apply for the job you told me about?

   B: No, I _____ take a few more classes and get more experience.

6. A: Did you know that I found an apartment on 45th Street? I _____
   move soon.

   B: That's a nice area. I _____ help you move if you like.

   A: Great! I'd really appreciate that.

7. A: Why can't you come to the party?

   B: We _____ be with my husband's family that weekend.

8. A: I have to leave. I don't have time to finish the dishes.

   B: No problem. I _____ do them for you.

9. A: Do you want to go to the meeting together?

   B: Sure. I _____ meet you by the elevator in ten minutes.

EXERCISE 21 ▶ Grammar, speaking, and writing. (Chart 3-5)

Part I. <u>Underline</u> the future verbs. Then in groups, discuss the questions on page 76.

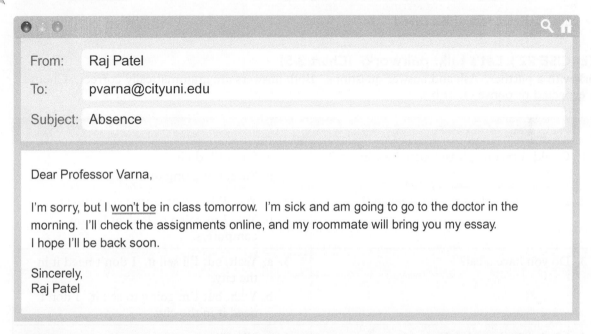

From: Raj Patel
To: pvarna@cityuni.edu
Subject: Absence

Dear Professor Varna,

I'm sorry, but I <u>won't be</u> in class tomorrow. I'm sick and am going to go to the doctor in the morning. I'll check the assignments online, and my roommate will bring you my essay.
I hope I'll be back soon.

Sincerely,
Raj Patel

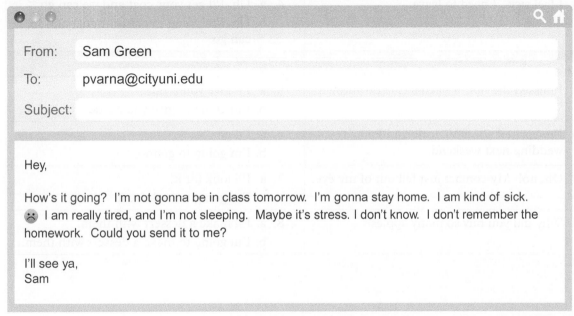

From: Sam Green
To: pvarna@cityuni.edu
Subject:

Hey,

How's it going? I'm not gonna be in class tomorrow. I'm gonna stay home. I am kind of sick. ☹ I am really tired, and I'm not sleeping. Maybe it's stress. I don't know. I don't remember the homework. Could you send it to me?

I'll see ya,
Sam

1. What differences do you notice between the two emails?
2. Which email do you think is better to send to a teacher?
3. Are there things in the second email that a teacher might not like?
4. What do you think are some features of an appropriate email? What are not? Make a list.
5. *Dear Professor …* is a form of address. Not all teachers are professors. What other forms of address are possible for writing to a teacher?
6. How much information do you think a teacher needs to have about an illness?

Part II. Write a formal email to your English teacher about missing class next week. Include these details.

- miss class on Monday
- sick
- check assignments with a friend

EXERCISE 22 ▶ Let's talk: pairwork. (Chart 3-5)
Work with a partner. Ask and answer questions. Both answers are grammatically correct. Choose the <u>expected</u> response (a. or b.).

PARTNER A	PARTNER B
1. Could someone please open the window?	1. a. Sure, I'll do it. b. Sure, I'm going to do it.
2. Do you have plans for the weekend?	2. a. Yes. I'll look at laptop computers. b. Yes. I'm going to look at laptop computers.
3. Do you have a car?	3. a. Yeah, but I'll sell it. I don't need it in the city. b. Yeah, but I'm going to sell it. I don't need it in the city.
4. I feel sick. I need to leave.	4. a. Uh, I'll get your coat and we can go. b. Uh, I'm going to get your coat and we can go.
PARTNER B	PARTNER A
5. I missed the bus. I need a ride downtown.	5. a. I'll give you a ride. b. I'm going to give you a ride.
6. I'm excited about Victoria and Peter's wedding next weekend.	6. a. I'll go too. b. I'm going to go too.
7. Oh, no! My contact just fell out of my eye.	7. a. I'll look for it. b. I'm going to look for it.
8. Why did you buy so many apples?	8. a. I'll make a dessert with them. b. I'm going to make a dessert with them.

EXERCISE 23 ▸ Warm-up. (Chart 3-6)

How certain is the speaker in each sentence? Write the percentage next to each sentence: 100%, 90%, or 50%.

What is going to happen to gasoline prices?

1. _____ Gas prices may rise.

2. _____ Maybe gas prices will rise.

3. _____ Gas prices will rise.

4. _____ Gas prices will probably rise.

5. _____ Gas prices are going to rise.

6. _____ Gas prices won't rise.

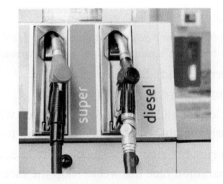

3-6 Certainty About the Future

100% sure	(a) I *will be* in class tomorrow. OR I *am going to be* in class tomorrow.	In (a): The speaker uses *will* or *be going to* because he feels sure about his future activity. He is stating a fact about the future.

90% sure	(b) Po *will probably be* in class tomorrow.
	OR
	Po *is probably going to be* in class tomorrow.
	
	(c) Anna *probably won't be* in class tomorrow.
	OR
	Anna *probably isn't going to be* in class tomorrow.
		In (b): The speaker uses *probably* to say that he expects Po to be in class tomorrow, but he is not 100% sure. He's almost sure, but not completely sure.
		Word order with *probably*:*
		(1) in a statement, as in (b):
		   helping verb + *probably*
		(2) with a negative verb, as in (c):
		   probably + *helping verb*

50% sure	(d) Ali *may come* to class tomorrow. OR Ali *may not come* to class tomorrow. I don't know what he's going to do.	*May* expresses a future possibility: maybe something will happen, and maybe it won't happen.** In (d): The speaker is saying that maybe Ali will come to class, or maybe he won't come to class. The speaker is guessing.
	(e) *Maybe* Ali *will come* to class, and *maybe* he *won't*. OR *Maybe* Ali *is going to come* to class, and *maybe* he *isn't*.	*Maybe* + *will/be going to* gives the same meaning as *may*. Examples (d) and (e) have the same meaning. *Maybe* comes at the beginning of a sentence.

*Probably is a midsentence adverb. See Chart 1-5, p. 14, for more information about the placement of midsentence adverbs.
**See Chart 7-3, p. 198, for more information about *may*.

EXERCISE 24 ▶ Grammar and speaking. (Chart 3-6)

For each situation, predict what probably will happen and what probably won't happen. Use either **will** or **be going to**. Include **probably** in your prediction.

1. Antonio is late to class almost every day. (be on time tomorrow? be late again?)

   → *Antonio probably won't be on time tomorrow. He'll probably be late again.* OR
   Antonio probably isn't going to be on time tomorrow. He's probably going to be late again.

2. Rosa has a terrible cold. She feels miserable.
   (go to work tomorrow? stay home and rest?)

3. Sami didn't sleep at all last night. He stayed up with his friends.
   (go to bed early tonight? stay up all night again tonight?)

4. Gina loves to run, but right now she has sore knees and a sore ankle.
   (run in the marathon race this week? skip the race?)

EXERCISE 25 ▶ Listening. (Chart 3-6)

Listen to the sentences. Decide the certainty for each one: 100%, 90%, or 50%.

My Day Tomorrow

Example: You will hear: The weather will be cold tomorrow.

   You will write: ___100%___

1. _____   3. _____   5. _____

2. _____   4. _____   6. _____

EXERCISE 26 ▶ Looking at grammar. (Chart 3-6)

Rewrite the sentences using the words in parentheses.

1. I may be late. (*maybe*) ___Maybe I will be late._____

2. Lisa may not get here. (*maybe*) _____

3. Maybe you will win the contest. (*may*) _____

4. The plane may land early. (*maybe*) _____

5. Maybe Sergio won't pass the class. (*may*) _____

EXERCISE 27 ▶ Let's talk: interview. (Chart 3-6)

Walk around the room. Take turns asking and answering the questions. Ask two students each question. Answer with **will**, **be going to**, or **may**. Use **probably** or **maybe** as appropriate.

Example: What will you do after class tomorrow?

   → *I'll probably go back to my apartment.* OR *I'm not sure. I may go to the bookstore.*

1. Where will you be tomorrow afternoon?
2. Where will you be next year?
3. What are you going to do on your next vacation?
4. Who will be the most famous celebrity next year?
5. What will a phone look like ten years from now?
6. What do you think will be the next big discovery in medicine?

EXERCISE 28 ▸ Reading, grammar, and speaking. (Charts 3-1 → 3-6)

Part I. Read the blog entry by co-author Stacy Hagen. Then answer the questions that follow.

BlackBookBlog

Do you know these words?
- discount
- insurance company
- brand
- advertising
- encourage

Money-Saving Tips for Students

If you are a student and do not live at home, the cost of living may surprise you. Life can be very expensive! Fortunately there are many ways to save money. If you search the phrase "students save money" on the internet, for example, you will find lots of useful tips. I'd like to share a few of my favorites with you.

1. **Ask about student discounts.**

   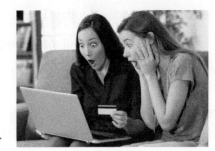

   Many businesses offer discounts to students. It is always a good idea to ask, "Do you have a student discount?" At the beginning of the school year, you will frequently find discounts from stores that sell clothes, computers, and housewares. In general, movie theaters offer a student discount year-round. Buses and trains usually give students a lower price. If you get good grades, some insurance companies will even give you a discount on your car insurance. Be sure you carry your student ID with you when you shop.

2. **Buy generic.**

   When you walk down a grocery store aisle, you will see a lot of different brands. Which one are you going to buy? How will you decide? One solution is to buy a generic brand. For example, let's say you like soft drinks. You can buy one that says *cola*. It doesn't have a special name. This is the generic product. Generics don't have advertising, so they will usually be cheaper.

3. **Don't shop when you are hungry!**

   This is a very simple tip. Research shows that if you shop when you are hungry, you will spend more money. Food looks much better on an empty stomach. It also helps to have a shopping list with you. If you get hungry when you are shopping, tell yourself that you will only buy the food on your list.

4. **Take care of your needs, not your wants.**

   It is important to separate needs from wants. Many things seem like needs, but they are actually just things you would like to have. Do you need to buy a cup of coffee from a coffee shop? You will save more money if you make it at home. Do you need to go to a sports event, or can you watch it on TV? Wants are nice, but they are also expensive.

   If you find these tips useful, I encourage you to look for more on the internet. You will probably find many more ways to save money. Good luck!

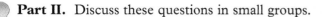

Part II. Discuss these questions in small groups.

1. What kind of student discounts are you already getting? What kind of discounts will you look for the next time you shop?
2. If you are at the store and see a cheaper brand that you don't know anything about and a more expensive brand that you already like, what are you going to buy and why?
3. Make a list of some of your wants and needs.
4. Do you have any shopping habits that you will change? List some things that you will and won't do to save money when you shop.
5. What do you, as a group, feel are the best ways to save money? Present a few of your suggestions to the class.

EXERCISE 29 ▸ Warm-up. (Chart 3-7)
Complete the sentences with your own words. What do you notice about the verb tenses and the words in green?

1. After I leave school today, I'm going to _____ .

2. Before I come to school tomorrow, I will _____ .

3. If I have time this weekend, I will _____ .

3-7	Expressing the Future in Time Clauses and *If*-Clauses

TIME CLAUSE (a) *Before I go to class tomorrow,* I'm going to eat breakfast. TIME CLAUSE (b) I'm going to eat breakfast *before I go to class tomorrow.*	In (a) and (b): *before I go to class tomorrow* is a future time clause. $\left. \begin{array}{l} \textbf{\textit{before}} \\ \textbf{\textit{after}} \\ \textbf{\textit{when}} \\ \textbf{\textit{as soon as}} \\ \textbf{\textit{until}} \\ \textbf{\textit{while}} \end{array} \right\}$ + *subject and verb* = a time clause
(c) *Before I go home tonight,* I'm going to stop at the market. (d) I'm going to eat dinner at 6:00 tonight. *After I eat dinner,* I'm going to study in my room. (e) I'll give Rita your message *when I see her.* (f) It's raining right now. *As soon as the rain stops,* I'm going to walk downtown. (g) I'll stay home *until the rain stops.* (h) *While you're at school tomorrow,* I'll be at work.	The simple present is used in a future time clause. ***Will*** and ***be going to*** are NOT used in a future time clause. INCORRECT: *Before I will go to class, I'm going to eat breakfast.* INCORRECT: *Before I am going to go to class tomorrow, I'm going to eat breakfast.* All of the example sentences (c) through (h) contain future time clauses.
(i) Maybe it will rain tomorrow. *If it rains tomorrow,* I'm going to stay home.	In (i): *If it rains tomorrow* is an ***if***-clause. ***if*** + *subject and verb* = an ***if***-clause When the meaning is future, the simple present (not ***will*** or ***be going to***) is used in an ***if***-clause.

EXERCISE 30 ▸ Looking at grammar. (Chart 3-7)
Choose the correct verbs.

1. Before   I'm going to return / (I return)   to my country next year, I'm going to finish my graduate degree in computer science.

2. My boss will review my work after she   will return / returns   from vacation next week.

3. I'll text you as soon as my plane   will land / lands.

4. I don't especially like my current job, but I'm going to stay with this company until

    I   find / will find   something better.

5. I need to find someone to water my vegetable garden when I

    am / will be   away next week.

6. If it   won't be / isn't   cold tomorrow, we'll go to the beach. If it

    is / will be   cold tomorrow, we'll go to a movie.

7. When you   will be / are   in Australia next month, are you going to explore the Great Barrier Reef?

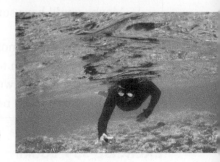

EXERCISE 31 ▸ Looking at grammar. (Chart 3-7)
Use the given verbs to complete the sentences. Use **be going to** for the future.

To-Do List

1. *take / reread*   I _'m going to reread_ the textbook before I ___take___ the final exam next month.

2. *clean / finish*   Tim _____ his desk as soon as he _____
    class.

3. *make / go*   Before I _____ to my job interview next week, I _____
    _____ a list of questions I want to ask about the company.

4. *visit / fix*   Tom _____ the leak in his mom's roof when he
    _____ her next week.

5. *look for / find*   I _____ cell phones online until I _____
    a good deal.★

6. *wash / stop*   If the rain _____, Dan _____ his car.

7. *work / get*   If Eva _____ home early, we _____ in our
    vegetable garden.

★Time clauses beginning with **until** usually <u>follow</u> the main clause.
    Usual: I'm going to look for cell phones online **until** I *find a good deal.*
    Possible but less usual: **Until** I *find a good deal,* I'm going to look for cell phones online.

EXERCISE 32 ▸ Let's talk: pairwork. (Chart 3-7)

Work with a partner. Take turns saying a sentence. Your partner will add a sentence using *if*. Pay special attention to the verb in the *if*-clause. Share some of your partner's answers.

Example: Maybe you'll go downtown tomorrow.
PARTNER A: Maybe you'll go downtown tomorrow.
PARTNER B: If I **go** downtown tomorrow, I'm going to look at laptop computers.

PARTNER A	PARTNER B
1. Maybe you'll have some free time tomorrow.	1. Maybe you'll be tired tonight.
2. Maybe it'll rain tomorrow.	2. Maybe you won't be tired tonight.
3. Maybe it won't rain tomorrow.	3. Maybe it'll be nice tomorrow.
4. Maybe the teacher will be absent next week.	4. Maybe we won't have class on Monday.
5. Maybe you'll win a new car tomorrow.	5. Maybe you'll win a lot of money next month.
	Change roles.

EXERCISE 33 ▸ Looking at grammar. (Chart 3-7)

Look at Sue's smartphone calendar. She has a busy morning. Make sentences using the words in parentheses and the given information. Use *be going to* for the future.

A Busy Day

1. (*after*)   go to the dentist \ pick up groceries
    → *After Sue goes to the dentist, she is going to pick up groceries.*
2. (*before*)   go to the dentist \ pick up groceries
3. (*before*)   have lunch with Hiro \ pick up groceries
4. (*after*)   have lunch with Hiro \ pick up groceries
5. (*before*)   have lunch with Hiro \ take her father to his doctor's appointment

●●○○○ 🔋	10:48	✈ ❋ ■□
‹ April	☰	Q +

Thu., Apr. 11	
9:00	dentist
10:00	groceries
11:00	lunch with Hiro
12:00	Dr.'s appt. – Dad

EXERCISE 34 ▸ Looking at grammar. (Chapters 1, 2 and Chart 3-7)

Complete each sentence with a form of the words in parentheses. Pay attention to the time words. Use a form of *be going to* for the future.

1. Before Aiden (*go*) _____ goes _____ to bed, he always (*brush*) _____ brushes _____ his teeth.

2. Before Aiden (*go*) _____ to bed later tonight, he (*brush*) _____
   his teeth.

3. Before Aiden (*go*) _____ to bed last night,
   he (*brush*) _____ his teeth.

4. While Aiden (*take*) _____
   a shower last night, the smoke alarm (*go off*)
   _____ .

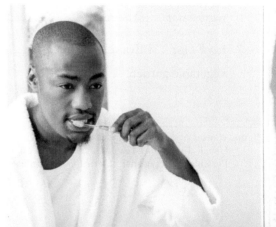
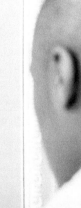

5. As soon as the smoke alarm (*go off*) _____ last night, Aiden (*jump*)

    _____ out of the shower to turn it off.

6. As soon as Aiden (*get*) _____ up tomorrow morning, he (*fix*)

    _____ the smoke alarm.

7. Aiden always (*fix*) _____ things as soon as they (*break*) _____ .

EXERCISE 35 ▶ Warm-up. (Chart 3-8)
Which sentences express future time?

1. I'm catching a train tonight.
2. I'm going to take the express train.
3. The trip will only take an hour.
4. My parents are picking me up.

3-8 Using the Present Progressive to Express Future Time

(a) Tim *is going to come* to the party tomorrow. (b) Tim *is coming* to the party tomorrow.	The present progressive can be used to express future time. Each pair of example sentences has the same meaning.
(c) We*'re going to go* to a movie tonight. (d) We*'re going* to a movie tonight. (e) I*'m going to stay* home this evening. (f) I*'m staying* home this evening. (g) Ann *is going to fly* to Miami next week. (h) Ann *is flying* to Miami next week.	The present progressive describes *definite plans for the future, plans that were made before the moment of speaking.* A future meaning for the present progressive is indicated either by future time words (e.g., *tomorrow*) or by the situation.*
(i) You*'re going to laugh* when you hear this joke. (j) INCORRECT: *You're laughing when you hear this joke.*	The present progressive is NOT used for predictions about the future. In (i): The speaker is predicting a future event. In (j): The present progressive is not possible; laughing is a prediction, not a planned future event.

*COMPARE: Present situation: *Look! Mary's coming. Do you see her?*
              Future situation: *Are you planning to come to the party? Mary's coming. So is Alex.*

EXERCISE 36 ▶ Looking at grammar. (Chart 3-8)
Complete the conversations with the correct form of the present progressive. Discuss whether the present progressive expresses present or future time.

1. A: What (*you, do*) _____*are you doing*_____ tomorrow afternoon?

   B: I (*go*) _____*am going*_____ to the mall. How about you? What (*you, do*)

     _____ tomorrow afternoon?

   A: I (*go*) _____ to a movie with Dan. After the movie, we (*go*)

     _____ out to dinner. Would you like to meet us for dinner?

   B: No, thanks. I can't. I (*meet*) _____ my son for dinner.

2. A: What (*you, major*) _____ in?

   B: I (*major*) _____ in engineering.

   A: What courses (*you, take*) _____ next semester?

   B: I (*take*) _____ English, math, and physics.

3. A: Stop! Paula! What (*you, do*) _____ ?

   B: I (*cut*) _____ my hair, Mom.

EXERCISE 37 ▶ Listening. (Chart 3-8)
Listen to the conversation and write the words you hear.

Going on Vacation

A: I _____ on vacation tomorrow.
                        1

B: Where _____ you _____ ?
            2   3

A: To San Francisco.

B: How are you getting there? _____ you _____ or _____ your car?
                               4   5   6

A: I _____. I want to be at the airport by 7:00 tomorrow morning.
        7

B: Do you need a ride to the airport?

A: No, thanks. I _____ a taxi. What about you? Are you planning to go
                    8
   somewhere over vacation?

B: No. I _____ here.
          9

EXERCISE 38 ▶ Let's talk: pairwork. (Chart 3-8)
Work with a partner. Tell each other your plans. Use the present progressive.

Example:
PARTNER A: What are your plans for this evening?
PARTNER B: I'm staying home. How about you?
PARTNER A: I'm going to a coffee shop to work on my paper for a while. Then I'm meeting some
            friends for a movie.

What are your plans for …

1. the rest of today?   3. this coming weekend?
2. tomorrow?   4. next month?

EXERCISE 39 ▶ Warm-up. (Chart 3-9)
Choose all the possible completions.

1. Soccer season begins _____.
   a. today   b. next week   c. yesterday

2. The mall opens _____.
   a. next Monday   b. tomorrow   c. today

3. There is a party _____ .
    a. last week   b. tonight   c. next weekend

4. The baby cries _____ .
    a. every night   b. tomorrow night   c. in the evenings

3-9   Using the Simple Present to Express Future Time

(a) My plane *arrives* at 7:35 *tomorrow evening*.	The simple present can express future time when events are on a definite schedule or timetable.
(b) Tim's new job *starts* next week.	
(c) The semester *ends* in two more weeks.	Only a few verbs are used in the simple present to express future time. The most common are ***arrive, leave, start, begin, end, finish, open, close, be***.
(d) There *is* a meeting at ten *tomorrow morning*.	
(e) INCORRECT: *I wear my new suit to the wedding next week.* CORRECT: *I am wearing/am going to wear* my new suit to the wedding next week.	Most verbs CANNOT be used in the simple present to express future time. For example, in (e): The verb ***wear*** does not express an event on a schedule or timetable. It cannot be used in the simple present to express future time.

EXERCISE 40 ▸ Looking at grammar. (Charts 3-8 and 3-9)
Choose <u>all</u> the possible completions.

1. The concert _____ at eight tonight.
    a. begins   b. is beginning   c. is going to begin

2. I _____ seafood pasta for dinner tonight.
    a. make   b. am making   c. am going to make

3. I _____ to school tomorrow morning. I need the exercise.
    a. walk   b. am walking   c. am going to walk

4. The bus _____ at 8:15 tomorrow morning.
    a. leaves   b. is leaving   c. is going to leave

5. I _____ the championship game on TV at Jonah's house tomorrow.
    a. watch   b. am watching   c. am going to watch

6. The game _____ at 1:00 tomorrow afternoon.
    a. starts   b. is starting   c. is going to start

7. Alexa's plane _____ at 10:10 tomorrow morning.
    a. arrives   b. is arriving   c. is going to arrive

8. I can't pick her up tomorrow, so she _____ the airport bus into the city.
    a. takes   b. is taking   c. is going to take

9. Jonas _____ to several companies. He hopes to get a full-time job soon.
    a. applies   b. is applying   c. is going to apply

10. School _____ next Wednesday. I'm excited for vacation to begin.
    a. ends   b. is ending   c. is going to end

EXERCISE 41 ▸ Warm-up. (Chart 3-10)

Choose the scene that this sentence best describes: *He **is about to** fight a fire.*

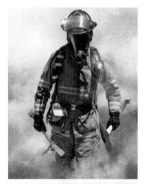

Picture A   Picture B

3-10 Immediate Future: Using *Be About To*	
(a) Ann is holding a suitcase, and she is wearing her coat. She *is about to leave* for the airport. (b) Shhh. The movie *is about to begin*.	The idiom ***be about to do something*** expresses an activity that will happen *in the immediate future*, usually within minutes or seconds. In (a): Ann is going to leave sometime in the next few minutes. In (b): The movie is going to start in the next few minutes.

EXERCISE 42 ▸ Let's talk. (Chart 3-10)

Make sentences with ***be about to***. Work in pairs, in small groups, or as a class.

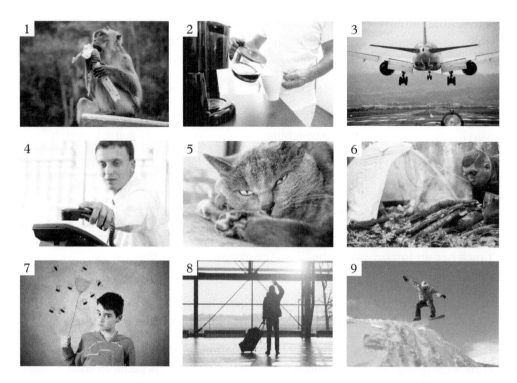

EXERCISE 43 ▸ Warm-up. (Chart 3-11)

Choose <u>all</u> the possible completions for each sentence.

1. Fifteen years from now, my wife and I will retire and _____ all over the world.
   a. will travel
   b. travel
   c. traveling
   d. going to travel
   e. are traveling
   f. traveled

2. I opened the door and _____ my friend to come in.
   a. will invite
   b. invite
   c. inviting
   d. am going to invite
   e. am inviting
   f. invited

3-11 Parallel Verbs

(a) Jim `makes` his bed `and` `cleans` up his room every morning. (b) Anita *called* and *told* me about her new job.	Often a subject has two verbs that are connected by **and**. We say that the two verbs are parallel: V + **and** + V *makes and cleans* = parallel verbs
(c) Ann *is cooking* dinner *and (is)* *talking* on the phone at the same time. (d) I *will stay* home *and (will)* *study* tonight. (e) I *am going to stay* home *and (am going to)* *study* tonight. NOT PARALLEL: *I am going to stay home and will study tonight.*	It is not necessary to repeat a helping verb (an auxiliary verb) when two verbs are the same tense and form and are connected by **and**.

EXERCISE 44 ▸ Looking at grammar. (Chart 3-11)

Complete each sentence with the correct form of the verbs in parentheses. More than one answer may be possible.

Work Woes

1. When I (*get*) _____ to work yesterday, a new employee (*stream*) _____ a movie and (*text*) _____ on her phone. That is not a good way to start!

2. My favorite manager is going to leave soon. She (*move*) _____ to San Francisco and (*work*) _____ for a start-up company as soon as her son (*graduate*) _____ from high school.

3. My mom (*call*) _____ me every Monday morning at work and (*complain*) _____ about her neighbors and their noisy weekend parties.

4. Is the meeting (*start*) _____ or (*end*) _____? It's hard to tell. Our meetings never (*start*) _____ or (*end*) _____ on time, and there is a lot of wasted time.

5. While Stephen (*sit*) _____ outside and (*drink*) _____

   a cup of coffee during his lunch break yesterday, a bee (*land*) _____ on his wrist

   and (*sting*) _____ him. Paul (*drop*) _____ the cup and

   (*spill*) _____ coffee all over his pants.

6. I worked an 80-hour week! I'm beat.* After I (*get*) _____ home, I

   (*take*) _____ a hot bath and (*go*) _____ to bed.

EXERCISE 45 ▶ Looking at grammar. (Chapters 1 → 3 Review)
Complete each sentence with the correct form of the words in parentheses.

1. I usually (*ride*) __*ride*__ my bike to work in the morning, but it (*rain*)

   _____ when I left my house early this morning, so I (*take*) _____

   the bus. After I (*get*) _____ to work, I (*find*) _____ out** that my briefcase
   was still on the bus.

2. A: Are you going to take the kids to the amusement park tomorrow morning?

   B: Yes. It (*open*) _____ at 10:00. If we (*leave*) _____ here at 9:30, we'll get
      there at 9:55. The kids can be the first ones in the park.

3. A: Ouch! I (*cut*) _____ my finger. It (*bleed*) _____!

   B: Put pressure on it. I (*get*) _____ some antibiotics and a bandage.

   A: Thanks.

4. A: Your phone (*ring*) _____.

   B: I (*know*) _____.

   A: (*you, want*) _____ me to get it?

   B: No.

   A: Why don't you want to answer your phone?

   B: I (*answer, never*) _____ during dinner.

5. A: Look! There (*be*) _____ a police car behind us. Its lights (*flash*) _____.

   B: I (*know*) _____. I (*know*) _____. I (*see*) _____ it.

   A: What (*go*) _____ on? (*you, speed*) _____?

   B: No, I'm not. I (*drive*) _____ the speed limit.

   A: Oh, look. The police car (*pass*) _____ us.

   B: Whew!

---

be beat = be very, very tired; be exhausted

**find out* = discover; learn

EXERCISE 46 ▶ Listening and speaking. (Chapters 1 → 3 Review)

Part I. Complete the sentences with the words you hear.

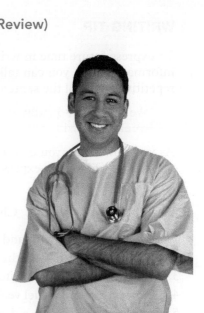

You will find love soon.

At a Chinese Restaurant

A: OK, let's all open our fortune cookies.

B: What _____ your cookie _____?

A: Mine says, "You _____ an unexpected gift."
Great! Are you planning to give me a gift soon?

B: Not that I know of. Mine says, "Your life _____ long and happy." Good.
I _____ a long life.

C: Mine says, "A smile _____ all communication problems." Well, that's
good! After this, when I _____ someone, _____ just
_____ at them.

D: My fortune is this: "If you _____ hard, you _____ successful."

A: Well, it _____ like all of us _____ good luck in the future!

Part II. Work in small groups. Together, write a fortune for each person in your group. Share a
few of the fortunes with the class.

EXERCISE 47 ▶ Check your knowledge. (Chapters 1 → 3 Review)
Correct the verb errors.

My Cousin Pablo

1. I want to tell you about Pablo. He *is* my cousin.

2. He comes here four years ago.

3. Before he came here, he study biology in Chile.

4. He leaves Chile and move here.

5. Then he went to New York and stay there for three years.

6. He graduates from New York University.

7. Now he study for his medical degree.

8. After he finish his medical degree, he return to Chile.

EXERCISE 48 ▸ Reading, grammar, and writing. (Chapter 3)

Part I. Read the social media post. <u>Underline</u> the verbs that express the future.

TRAVEL

A Weekend in Nashville   *November 3*

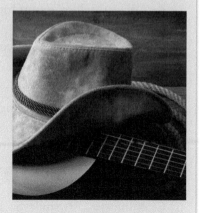

    My friend Sara and I <u>are taking</u> a trip to Nashville, Tennessee, soon. Nashville is the home of country music, and Sara loves country music. She wants to go to several shows. Nashville has more than 160 places to hear live music. Many country music singers become famous in Nashville. I don't know anything about country music, but I'm looking forward to going. We're leaving Friday evening as soon as Sara gets off work. We will be away for a week. We're going to take the train. It's a 14-hour trip, so we will sleep for part of the time. Sara has a cousin in Nashville. We are going to try to visit her, but it's possible she will be out of town. We are getting back on Sunday night because we both need to work on Monday. Sara and I are excited about our first trip to Nashville.

Part II. Imagine that you have a week's vacation. You can go anywhere you want. Think of a place you would like to visit, and write a paragraph to describe your plans. Use these questions as a guide. Remember to add variety by using different future verb forms and to use parallel verbs when appropriate.

1. Where and how are you going?
2. When are you leaving?
3. Who are you going with, or are you traveling alone?
4. Where are you staying?
5. Are you visiting anyone? Who?
6. How long are you staying there?
7. When are you getting back?

WRITING TIP

To express future time in writing, *will* is more common than other future forms. However, in informal writing, you can talk about the future in different ways to add interest. Look at how repetitive and dull the sentences from the reading become when only the verb *will* is used:

> We will leave Friday evening as soon as Sara gets off work. We will be away for two weeks. We will take the train. It's a 14-hour trip, so we will sleep part of the time.

As you now know, you can use not only *will* but also *be going to* and even the simple present or present progressive to express future time. These verbs will add more variety to your writing.

Part III. Edit your writing. Check for the following:

1. ☐ correct forms of **will** and **be going to**
2. ☐ use of some variety in the verb forms to express the future
3. ☐ use of simple present with time and *if*-clauses, where appropriate
4. ☐ correct use of parallel verbs
5. ☐ correct spelling (use a dictionary or spell-check)

▪▪▪▪▪ For digital resources, go to the Pearson Practice English app.

Present Perfect and Past Perfect

PRETEST: What do I already know?

Write "C" if the **boldfaced** words are correct and "I" if they are incorrect.

1. _____ **Have** you ever **eaten** something really unusual? (Charts 4-1 and 4-2)

2. _____ I **have** just **finish** my homework. (Chart 4-3)

3. _____ My mom **has** recently **become** the bank manager. (Chart 4-3)

4. _____ Eva and Julia have started kindergarten **yet**. (Chart 4-3)

5. _____ Food prices **have increased** several times. (Chart 4-3)

6. _____ William **has worked** as an auto mechanic since he **finished** college. (Chart 4-4)

7. _____ My grandfather **has died** in 1990. (Chart 4-5)

8. _____ Max **has been playing** video games for several hours. (Chart 4-6)

9. _____ Katrina **has been texting** since she woke up. (Chart 4-6)

10. _____ We **have been staying** at that hotel three times. (Chart 4-7)

11. _____ By the time the movie **finished**, half of the audience **had gone** home. (Chart 4-8)

EXERCISE 1 ▸ Warm-up. (Chart 4-1)

Do you know the past participle form of these verbs? Complete the chart. What is the difference between the past participle forms in items 1–4 and 5–8?

SIMPLE FORM	SIMPLE PAST	PAST PARTICIPLE
1. help	helped	_helped_
2. work	worked	_worked_
3. stay	stayed	_____
4. visit	visited	_____
5. eat	ate	_eaten_
6. have	had	_had_
7. write	wrote	_____
8. begin	began	_____

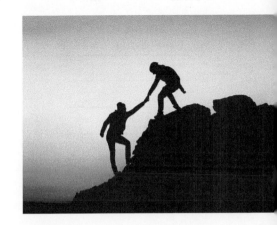

4-1 Past Participle

This chapter introduces the present perfect and past perfect tenses. In order to form these verbs, you need to know *the past participle forms*. The past participle is one of the principal parts of a verb. (See Appendix A-1.)

	SIMPLE FORM	SIMPLE PAST	PAST PARTICIPLE	
REGULAR VERBS	finish look stop try use wait	finished looked stopped tried used waited	**finished** **looked** **stopped** **tried** **used** **waited**	The past participle of regular verbs is the same as the simple past form: both end in *-ed*.
IRREGULAR VERBS	be come do find go get have know make say see take tell	was/were came did found went got had knew made said saw took told	**been** **come** **done** **found** **gone** **got/gotten** **had** **known** **made** **said** **seen** **taken** **told**	Many common verbs have irregular past forms. The verbs in the list are the most common irregular verbs. See Appendix A-2 or the inside back cover for a more complete list of irregular verbs.

EXERCISE 2 ▸ Looking at grammar. (Chart 4-1)

Part I. Write the simple past and the past participle of the <u>regular</u> (*-ed*) verbs in the box.

be	die	know	read	teach
✓call	do	leave	speak	think
come	finish	move	study	walk

SIMPLE FORM	SIMPLE PAST	PAST PARTICIPLE
1. _____call_____	_____called_____	_____called_____
2. _____	_____	_____
3. _____	_____	_____
4. _____	_____	_____
5. _____	_____	_____
6. _____	_____	_____

Part II. Write the simple past and the past participle of the <u>irregular</u> verbs in the box.

SIMPLE FORM	SIMPLE PAST	PAST PARTICIPLE
7. _____*be*_____	_____*was, were*_____	_____*been*_____
8. _____	_____	_____
9. _____	_____	_____
10. _____	_____	_____
11. _____	_____	_____
12. _____	_____	_____
13. _____	_____	_____
14. _____	_____	_____
15. _____	_____	_____

EXERCISE 3 ▸ Pairwork. (Chart 4-1)
Work with a partner. Give the past tense and past participle forms of the verb that your partner says.

PARTNER A: (*book open*) **PARTNER B:** (*book closed*)	**PARTNER B:** (*book open*) **PARTNER A:** (*book closed*)
1. give (*gave, given*)	8. say (*said, said*)
2. text (*texted, texted*)	9. begin (*began, begun*)
3. leave (*left, left*)	10. pay (*paid, paid*)
4. drive (*drove, driven*)	11. delete (*deleted, deleted*)
5. rent (*rented, rented*)	12. begin (*began, begun*)
6. forget (*forgot, forgotten*)	13. marry (*married, married*)
7. take (*took, taken*)	14. tell (*told, told*)

EXERCISE 4 ▸ Warm-up: pairwork. (Chart 4-2)
Work with a partner. Take turns asking and answering questions. Use the words in the box.

bought a boat	flown a drone	grown your own vegetables
climbed a tree	forgotten your age	ridden on a motorcycle

PARTNER A: Have you ever _____?
PARTNER B: Yes, I have. OR No, I've never _____.

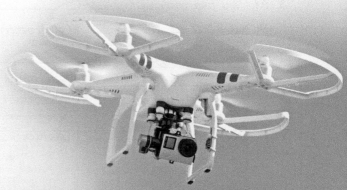

4-2 Introduction to the Present Perfect: Unspecified Time with *Ever* and *Never*

(a) — *Have* you *ever lost* your ID*? — No, I *have never lost* my ID. (b) — *Has* it *ever snowed* in your hometown? — No, it *has never snowed* in my hometown.	The PRESENT PERFECT is frequently used to express some *unspecified or unknown time in the past*. **Ever** and **never** are examples of time words that do not give a specific time. **ever** = in your lifetime; from the time you were born to the present moment. In the (a) and (b) responses, the speaker uses **never** to say, "No, I haven't lost my ID from the time I was born to the present moment," and, "No, it hasn't snowed in my hometown from the time I was born to the present moment." QUESTION: **have/has** + *subject* + **ever** + *past participle* NEGATIVE: **have/has** + **never** + *past participle*
(c) Has Jon *ever* met your family? — No, *he has not met* my family. No, he*'s not met* my family. No, he *has not*. No, he *hasn't*. — Yes, he *has met* my family. OR Yes, he *has*.	Note other ways to answer a question with **ever**. NEGATIVE: **have/has** + **not** + *past participle* NEGATIVE CONTRACTIONS: **have** + **not** = **haven't** **has** + **not** = **hasn't** AFFIRMATIVE STATEMENT: **have/has** + *past participle* CONTRACTED FORMS: *I've, You've, He's, She's, It's, We've, They've*

*ID = identification

EXERCISE 5 ▸ Looking at grammar. (Charts 4-1 and 4-2)

Complete the conversations. Use the present perfect form of the verbs in parentheses.

Unusual Experiences

1. A: (*you, see, ever*) _____Have you ever seen_____ a ghost?

   B: No, I ___haven't___. I (*see, never*) ___have never seen___ a ghost.

2. A: (*you, eat, ever*) _____ an insect?

   B: No, I _____. I (*eat, never*) _____ an insect.

3. A: (*you, find, ever*) _____ a gold coin?

   B: No, I _____. I (*find, never*) _____ a gold coin.

4. A: (*you, talk, ever*) _____ to a movie star?

   B: No, I _____. I (*talk, never*) _____ to a movie star.

5. A: (*you, go, ever*) _____ for a ride in a spaceship?

   B: No, I _____. I (*go, never*) _____ for a ride in a spaceship.

EXERCISE 6 ▶ Grammar and speaking. (Charts 4-1 and 4-2)

Complete the sentences with the correct form of the verbs in parentheses. Then choose a true answer for you. Share your answers with a partner. Use these forms: *I have* or *I have never.*

1. Have you ever (*see*) _____ snow?   yes   no

2. Have you ever (*fly*) _____ in a small plane?   yes   no

3. Have you ever (*run*) _____ for an hour without stopping?   yes   no

4. Have you ever (*do*) _____ volunteer work?   yes   no

5. Have you ever (*tear*) _____ a muscle?   yes   no

6. Have you ever (*have*) _____ a bad experience on a plane?   yes   no

    a muscle

7. Have you ever (*fall*) _____ out of a tree?   yes   no

8. Have you ever (*feel*) _____ so embarrassed that your face got hot?   yes   no

9. Have you ever (*speak*) _____ to a famous person?   yes   no

10. Have you ever (*win*) _____ a contest?   yes   no

EXERCISE 7 ▶ Let's talk: interview. (Charts 4-1 and 4-2)

Interview your classmates. Make questions using the present perfect form of the verbs. Share some of your information with the class.

1. you \ ever \ cut \ your own hair _____

2. you \ ever \ catch \ a big fish _____

3. you \ ever \ take care of \ an animal _____

4. you \ ever \ lose \ something very important _____

5. you \ ever \ sit \ on a bee _____

6. you \ ever \ break \ your arm or your leg _____

7. you \ ever \ throw \ a ball \ and \ hit \ a window _____

8. you \ ever \ swim \ in the Atlantic Ocean _____

EXERCISE 8 ▶ Warm-up. (Chart 4-3)

Choose the correct answer for each sentence.

1. Tyler has rented a small house _____.   a. last week   b. recently

2. I have seen it _____.   a. already   b. two days ago

3. His parents haven't seen it _____.   a. yesterday   b. yet

4. I have been there _____.   a. twice   b. yesterday

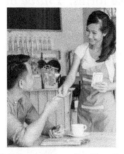

Erik has just eaten lunch.

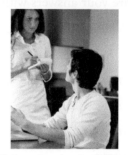

Ty hasn't eaten lunch yet.

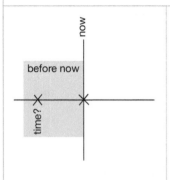	(a) Erik *has just eaten* lunch. (b) Jim *has recently changed* jobs.	The present perfect expresses an activity or situation that happened (or did not happen) *before now, at some unspecified or unknown time in the past.* As you learned in Chart 4-2, *ever* and *never* express an activity that occurred at an unknown time. Other common time words that express this idea are *just, recently, already,* and *yet.* In (a): Erik's lunch occurred before the present time. The exact time is not mentioned; it is unimportant or unknown.
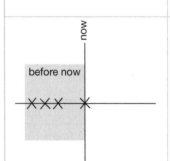	(c) Pete *has eaten* at that restaurant *many times.* (d) I *have eaten* there *twice.*	An activity may be repeated two, several, or more times *before now, at unspecified times in the past,* as in (c) and (d). Use of the present perfect can indicate that the activity may happen again.
	(e) Pele *has already left*. OR Pele *has left already.*	In (e): **Already** is used in affirmative statements. It can come after the helping verb or at the end of the sentence. Idea of **already:** Something happened before now, before this time.
	(f) Ty *hasn't eaten yet*.	In (f): **Yet** is used in negative statements and comes at the end of the sentence. Idea of **yet:** Something did not happen before now (up to this time), but it may happen in the future.
	(g) *Have* you *already left*? *Have* you *left already*? *Have* you *left yet*?	In (g): Both **yet** and **already** can also be used in questions. NOTE: Sometimes the speaker doesn't use a time word. It is implied. *Ty hasn't eaten.* = *Ty hasn't eaten yet.*

EXERCISE 9 ▸ Looking at grammar. (Chart 4-3)

Complete each question with the correct form of the verb in parentheses.

New Parents

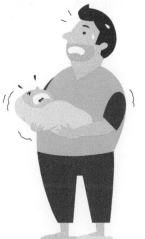

1. Has Richard (*hold*) _____ held _____ the baby a lot yet?

2. Has Lori (*give*) _____ the baby a bath already?

3. Has Richard (*change*) _____ a diaper yet?

4. Has Lori (*take*) _____ some pictures of the baby already?

5. Has Richard (*get*) _____ up in the middle of the night yet?

6. Has Lori (*have*) _____ problems sleeping already?

7. Has Richard (*feel*) _____ tired during the day yet?

8. Has the baby (*sleep*) _____ through the night already?

EXERCISE 10 ▸ Looking at grammar. (Chart 4-3)

Choose <u>all</u> the possible answers for each question. Work in small groups and then discuss your answers as a class.

SITUATION 1: Sara is at home. At 12:00 P.M., the phone rang. It was Sara's friend from high school. They had a long conversation, and Sara hung up the phone at 12:59. It is now 1:00. Which sentences describe the situation?

   a. Sara has just hung up the phone.
   b. She has hung up the phone already.
   c. The phone has just rung.
   d. Sara hasn't finished her conversation yet.

SITUATION 2: Mr. Peters is in bed. He became sick with the flu eight days ago. Mr. Peters isn't sick very often. The last time he had the flu was one year ago. Which sentences describe the situation?

   a. Mr. Peters has been sick for a year.
   b. He hasn't gotten well yet.
   c. He has just gotten sick.
   d. He has already had the flu.
   e. He hasn't had the flu before.

SITUATION 3: Rob is at work. His boss, Rosa, needs a report. She sees Rob working on it at his desk. She's in a hurry, and she's asking Rob questions. What questions is she going to ask him?

   a. Have you finished?
   b. Have you finished yet?
   c. Have you finished already?
   d. Have you already finished?

EXERCISE 11 ▶ Looking at grammar. (Chart 4-3)

Look at Andy's smartphone calendar. Write answers to the questions. Make complete sentences with **yet** and **already**.

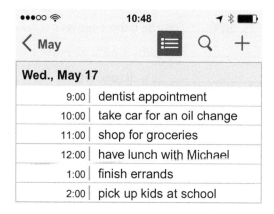

It is 11:55 A.M. right now.

1. Has Andy had his dentist appointment yet? _____Yes, he has had his dentist appointment already._____
   OR _Yes, he has already had his dentist appointment._____

2. Has Andy picked up his kids at school yet? _____

3. Has Andy taken his car for an oil change already? _____

4. Has Andy finished his errands yet? _____

5. Has Andy shopped for groceries already? _____

6. Has Andy had lunch with Michael yet? _____

EXERCISE 12 ▶ Listening. (Chart 4-3)

Both **is** and **has** can be contracted to **'s**. Listen to each sentence. Decide if the contracted verb is **is** or **has**. Before you begin, you may want to check your understanding of these words: *order, waiter.*

At a Restaurant

Examples: You will hear: My order's taking a long time.
            You will choose: (is)   has

            You will hear: My order's already taken a long time.
            You will choose: is   (has)

1. is   has   4. is   has

2. is   has   5. is   has

3. is   has   6. is   has

EXERCISE 13 ▸ Warm-up. (Chart 4-4)

Choose the correct sentence (a. or b.) to describe each situation.

1. It's 10:00 A.M. Layla has been at the bus stop since 9:50.
   a. She is still there.   b. The bus picked her up.

2. Toshi has lived in the same apartment for 30 years.
   a. After 30 years, he moved somewhere else.   b. He still lives there.

4-4 Present Perfect with *Since* and *For*

10:00 A.M. ⟶ now	(a) I've been in class *since ten o'clock this morning*.	The present perfect tense is used in sentences with **since** and **for** to express situations that began in the past and continue to the present.
	(b) We have known Ben for *ten years*. We met him ten years ago. We still know him today. We are friends.	In (a): Class started at ten. I am still in class now, at the moment of speaking. INCORRECT: *I am in class since ten o'clock this morning.*

Since

(c) I *have been* here { since eight o'clock. since Tuesday. since 2009. since yesterday. since last month.	**Since** is followed by the mention of a *specific point in time*: an hour, a day, a month, a year, etc. **Since** expresses the idea that something began at a specific time in the past and continues to the present.

(d) CORRECT: I *have lived* here since May.* CORRECT: I *have been* here since May. (e) INCORRECT: *I am living here since May.* (f) INCORRECT: *I live here since May.* (g) INCORRECT: *I lived here since May.* (h) INCORRECT: *I was here since May.*	Notice the incorrect sentences: In (e): The present progressive is NOT used. In (f): The simple present is NOT used. In (g) and (h): The simple past is NOT used.

MAIN CLAUSE (present perfect)	SINCE-CLAUSE (simple past)	**Since** may also introduce a time clause (i.e., a subject and verb may follow **since**).
(i) I *have lived* here	since I *was* a child.	Notice in the examples: The present perfect is used in the main clause; the simple past is used in the *since*-clause.
(j) Al *has met* many people	since he *came* here.	

For

(k) I *have been* here { for ten minutes. for two hours. for five days. for about three weeks. for almost six months. for many years. for a long time.	**For** is followed by the mention of a *length of time*: two minutes, three hours, four days, five weeks, etc.).

*Also correct: *I have been living* here since May. See Chart 4-6 for a discussion of the present perfect progressive.

EXERCISE 14 ▶ Looking at grammar. (Chart 4-4)
Complete the sentences with *since* or *for*.

Amy has been here …

1. _____for_____ two months.
2. _____since_____ September.
3. _____ yesterday.
4. _____ the term started.
5. _____ a couple of hours.
6. _____ fifteen minutes.

Ms. Ellis has worked as a substitute teacher …

11. _____ school began.
12. _____ last year.
13. _____ 2008.
14. _____ about a year.
15. _____ September.
16. _____ a long time.

The Smiths have been married …

7. _____ two years.
8. _____ last May.
9. _____ five days.
10. _____ a long time.

I've known about Sonia's engagement …

17. _____ almost four months.
18. _____ the beginning of the year.
19. _____ the first of January.
20. _____ yesterday.

EXERCISE 15 ▶ Looking at grammar. (Chart 4-4)
Complete the sentences with information about yourself.

1. I've been in this building
   - since _nine o'clock this morning_____ .
   - for _27 minutes_____ .

2. We've been in class
   - since _____ .
   - for _____ .

3. I've been in this city/town
   - since _____ .
   - for _____ .

4. I've had an ID card
   - since _____ .
   - for _____ .

5. I've had this book
   - since _____ .
   - for _____ .

6. I've been a student
   - since _____ .
   - for _____ .

EXERCISE 16 ▶ Looking at grammar. (Chart 4-4)

Complete each sentence with the present perfect form of the given verb.

A Talk-Show Host

Since 1995, Theresa, a talk-show host, ...

1. (*work*) _____has worked_____ for a TV station in London.

2. (*interview*) _____ hundreds of guests.

3. (*meet*) _____ many famous people.

4. (*find*) _____ out about their lives.

5. (*make*) _____ friends with celebrities.

6. (*become*) _____ a celebrity herself.

7. (*sign*) _____ lots of autographs.

8. (*shake*) _____ hands with thousands of people.

9. (*write*) _____ two books about how to interview people.

10. (*think*) _____ a lot about the best ways to help people feel comfortable on her show.

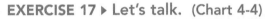

EXERCISE 17 ▶ Let's talk. (Chart 4-4)

Your teacher will ask questions. One student will answer with **since**. Another student will use that information and answer with **for**. Only the teacher's book is open.

Example:

To STUDENT A: How long have you been in this room?
  STUDENT A: I've been in this room **since** (10:00).
To STUDENT B: How long has (*Student A*) been in this room?
  STUDENT B: She/He has been in this room **for** (15 minutes).

1. How long have you known me?
2. How long have you been up* today?
3. Where do you live? How long have you lived there?
4. Who has a cell phone? How long have you had your phone?
5. Who has a bike? How long have you had it?
6. How long have you been in this building today?
7. Who is wearing something new? What is it? How long have you had it/them?
8. Who is married? How long have you been married?

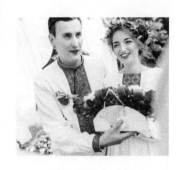

---

*be up = be awake and out of bed

EXERCISE 18 ▸ Looking at grammar. (Chart 4-4)

Put brackets [ ] around the *since*-clauses. Then choose the correct form of the verbs.

Car Problems

1. Otto   had / (has had)   a lot of problems with his car [ever since* he (bought) / has bought   it.]

2. Ever since Tina   took / has taken   her car in for repairs, it   didn't run / hasn't run   properly.

3. Thomas's car   had / has had   engine problems since he   had / has had   an accident.

4. Ever since my friend   changed / has changed   the oil in my car,

    I   noticed / have noticed   smoke in the engine.

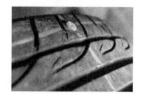

5. My tire   had / has had   a slow leak ever since I   drove / have driven

    through a construction area. Maybe it has a nail in it.

EXERCISE 19 ▸ Let's talk: pairwork. (Charts 4-1, 4-2, and 4-4)

With a partner, take turns asking and answering questions. Begin questions with **How long have you** and the present perfect. Answer with **since, for,** or **never** and the present perfect.

Example: have a pet
PARTNER A: How long have you had a pet?
PARTNER B: I've had (*a cat, a dog, a bird, etc.*) for two years/since my 18th birthday. OR
                   I've never had a pet.

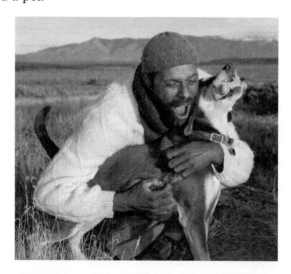

PARTNER A	PARTNER B
1. live in (*this area*)	1. wear glasses
2. study English	2. have a roommate
3. be in this class	3. have a pet
4. be at this school	4. be married
5. have long/short/medium-length hair	5. be interested in (*a particular subject*)
6. have a beard/mustache	6. want to be (*a particular profession*)
	Change roles.

Ever since is similar to *since*, but *ever* adds emphasis to the clause.

EXERCISE 20 ▸ Reading, grammar, and writing. (Charts 4-1 → 4-4)

Part I. Read the passage about Ellie. Underline the present perfect verbs.

Ellie

I'd like to tell you a little about Ellie. She has lived in Vancouver, Canada, for six months. She has studied English for five years. She has been at this school since September. She likes it here.

She has medium-length hair. She has never worn glasses, except sunglasses. She likes to wear hats. Of course, she has never had a mustache!

Ellie doesn't have a roommate, but she has a pet bird. She has had her bird for one month. His name is Howie, and he likes to sing.

She is interested in biology. She has been interested in biology since she was a child. She has never been married. She wants to be a doctor. She would like to become a doctor before she has a family.

Part II. Write about the person you interviewed in Exercise 19. You can ask additional questions to get more information. Use the passage about Ellie as an example.

EXERCISE 21 ▸ Looking at grammar. (Chart 4-4)

Complete the sentences with the correct form of the words in parentheses.

Life with My Host Family

1. I (know) _____have known_____ my host family ever since they (visit) _____visited_____ my parents three years ago.

2. Ever since I (get) _____ here, I (feel) _____ a little homesick.

3. My host family (move) _____ twice since I (begin) _____ school.

4. My host family is nice, but I can't wait to get home for vacation. I (see, not) _____ _____ my family since I (leave) _____ home nine months ago.

5. Ever since my host brother (meet) _____ his girlfriend, he (think, not) _____ _____ about anything or anyone else. He's in love.

6. My host family helped me find a car to buy, but I (have) _____ a lot of problems with it ever since I (buy) _____ it. My host mom is afraid it's a lemon.★

7. So far★★ I (enjoy) _____ my time with my host family.

★*a lemon* = a car with a lot of problems

★★*So far* + present perfect expresses situations that began in the past and continue to the present.

EXERCISE 22 ▸ Listening. (Charts 4-1 → 4-4)

Part I. When speakers use the present perfect in everyday speech, they often contract *have* and *has* with nouns. Listen to the sentences and notice the contractions.

Money Problems

1. Someone's taken my credit card.
2. Sorry. Your check's just bounced.
3. Both your credit cards've expired.
4. The bank's made an error again.
5. Checking fees've gone up for the third time.

Part II. Listen to the sentences. You will hear the contracted forms of the verbs. Complete the sentences with the non-contracted forms.

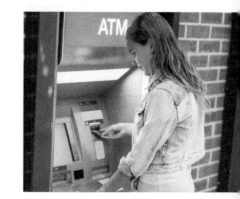

1. The cash machine _____ been out of service for two days.
2. I'm sorry. Your credit card _____ expired.
3. My checking account fees _____ increased a lot.
4. Someone _____ withdrawn money from your account.
5. Our new debit cards _____ gotten lost in the mail.

EXERCISE 23 ▸ Warm-up. (Chart 4-5)
Read the short conversation. Who is more likely to say the last sentence, Pam or Jen? Why?

> PAM: I've traveled around the world several times.
> JEN: I traveled around the world once.
> _____: I'm looking forward to my next trip.

4-5 Simple Past vs. Present Perfect

SIMPLE PAST (a) I *exercised* yesterday.	In (a): I exercised at a specific time in the past (*yesterday*).
PRESENT PERFECT (b) I *have* already *exercised*.	In (b): I exercised at an unspecified time in the past (*sometime before now*).
SIMPLE PAST (c) I *was* in Europe *last year / three years ago / in 2010 / in 2012 and 2016 / when I was ten years old.*	The simple past expresses an activity that occurred at a specific time (or times) in the past, as in (a) and (c).
PRESENT PERFECT (d) I *have been* in Europe *many times / several times / a couple of times / once / (no mention of time).*	The present perfect expresses an activity that occurred at an unspecified time (or times) in the past, as in (b) and (d). Use of the present perfect can indicate the activity may happen again. In (d), the speaker may return to Europe.
SIMPLE PAST (e) Ann *was* in Miami *for two weeks.* PRESENT PERFECT (f) Bob *has been* in Miami *for two weeks / since May 1st.*	In (e): In sentences where *for* is used in a time expression, the simple past expresses an activity that began and ended in the past. In (f): In sentences with *for* or *since*, the present perfect expresses an activity that began in the past and continues to the present.

EXERCISE 24 ▶ Looking at grammar. (Chart 4-5)

Look at the verbs in green. Are they simple past or present perfect? Check (✓) the correct time box.

	WE KNOW THE TIME	WE DON'T KNOW THE TIME
1. Ms. Parker has been in Tokyo many times. → *present perfect*	☐	☑
2. Ms. Parker was in Tokyo last week. → *simple past*	☑	☐
3. I've met Kaye's husband. He's a nice guy.	☐	☐
4. I met Kaye's husband at a party last week.	☐	☐
5. Mr. White was in the hospital last month.	☐	☐
6. Mr. White has been in the hospital many times.	☐	☐
7. I like to travel. I've been to more than 30 foreign countries.	☐	☐
8. I was in Morocco in 2008.	☐	☐

EXERCISE 25 ▶ Looking at grammar. (Chart 4-5)

Read the sentences about bikes and notice the verbs in green. Answer the questions that follow and explain your answers.

1. Ann had a fast bike.
   Sue has had a fast bike for two years.

   Who still has a fast bike? _____

2. Jill rode to work on her bike last week.
   Cathy has ridden to work on her bike since she got a new one.

   Who is still riding a bike to work? _____

3. In her lifetime, Aunt Alexa had several red bikes.
   In her lifetime, Grandma has had several red bikes.

   Who is still alive? _____ Who is dead? _____

4. Fernando has had several bikes in his lifetime.
   Jenny had a red bike when she was in elementary school.
   Keisha had a blue bike when she was a teenager.
   Chen had a gold bike when he lived and worked in Hong Kong.

   Who no longer has a bike?

   _____

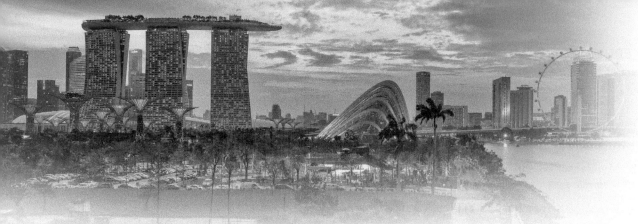

EXERCISE 26 ▸ **Looking at grammar.** (Chart 4-5)
Complete the sentences. Use the present perfect or the simple past form of the verbs in parentheses. NOTE: In informal spoken English, the simple past, rather than the present perfect, is sometimes used with **already**. In this exercise, however, practice using the present perfect with **already**.

1. A: Have you ever been to Singapore?

   B: Yes, I ___*have*___. I (be) ___*have been*___ to Singapore several times. In fact, I (be)
   ___*was*___ in Singapore last year.

2. A: Have you ever taken a tour of the city?

   B: Yes, I _____. I (take) _____ a few tours. Last year my wife and I (take)
   _____ a fun bike tour.

3. A: Are you going to book your flight this week?

   B: I (book, already) ___*have already booked*___ it. I (do) _____ it yesterday.

4. A: What African countries (you, visit) _____ so far?

   B: I (visit) _____ Kenya and Ethiopia. I (visit)
   _____ Kenya in 2002. I (be) _____ in Ethiopia last year.

5. A: When are you going to write about your trip in your blog?

   B: I (write, already) _____ it. I (write) _____
   it last night and (post) _____ it this morning.

6. A: (Romero, visit, ever) _____ family overseas?

   B: Yes, he _____. He (visit) _____ several times.

EXERCISE 27 ▸ **Let's talk: pairwork.** (Chart 4-5)
With a partner, ask and answer the questions. Use the present perfect or simple past.

Example:
PARTNER A: What countries have you been to?
PARTNER B: I've been to Norway and Finland.
PARTNER A: When were you in Norway?
PARTNER B: I was in Norway three years ago. How about you? What countries have you been to?
PARTNER A: I've never been to Norway or Finland, but I've been to … .

1. What countries have you been to? When were you in...?

2. Where are some interesting places you have lived? When did you live in...?

3. What are some interesting / unusual / scary things you have done in your lifetime? When did you...?

4. What are some helpful things (for a friend / your family / your community) you have done in your lifetime? When did you...?

EXERCISE 28 ▸ Listening. (Charts 2-3 and 4-5)
For each item, you will hear two complete sentences and then the beginning of a third sentence. Complete the third sentence with the past participle of the verb you heard in the first two sentences.

Example: You will hear: I eat vegetables every day. I ate vegetables for dinner last night. I have...

You will write: I have ___eaten___ vegetables every day for a long time.

1. Since Friday, I have _____ a lot of money.

2. All week, I have _____ big breakfasts.

3. Today, I have already _____ several emails.

4. I just finished dinner, and I have _____ a nice tip.

5. Since I was a teenager, I have _____ in late on weekends.

6. All my life, I have _____ very carefully.

7. Since I was little, I have _____ in the shower.

EXERCISE 29 ▸ Game. (Charts 4-1 → 4-5)
Work in groups:
1. On a piece of paper, write down two statements about yourself, one in the simple past tense and one in the present perfect tense.
2. Make one statement true and one statement false.
3. Say your sentences.
4. The other members of your group will try to guess which one is true.
5. Tell your group the answers after everyone has finished guessing.
The person with the most correct guesses at the end of the game is the winner.

Example:
STUDENT A: I've never cooked dinner.
          I saw a famous person last year.
STUDENT B: You've never cooked dinner. That is true.
          You saw a famous person last year. That is false.

EXERCISE 30 ▸ Warm-up. (Chart 4-6)
Complete the sentences with time information.

1. I am sitting at my desk right now. I have been sitting at my desk since _____.

2. I am looking at my book. I have been looking at my book for _____.

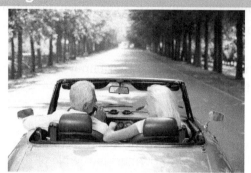

Al and Ann are in their car right now. They are driving home. It is now four o'clock.	The PRESENT PERFECT PROGRESSIVE talks about *how long* an activity has been in progress before now.
(a) They *have been driving* since two o'clock.	NOTE: Time expressions with **since**, as in (a), and **for**, as in (b), are frequently used with this tense.
(b) They *have been driving* for two hours. They will be home soon.	STATEMENT: **have/has + been + -ing**
(c) How long *have they been driving*?	QUESTION: **have/has + subject + been + -ing**

Present Progressive vs. Present Perfect Progressive

PRESENT PROGRESSIVE 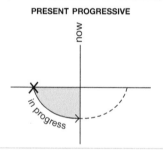	(d) Po *is sitting* in class right now.	The present progressive describes an activity that is in progress right now, as in (d). It does not discuss duration (length of time). *INCORRECT: Po has been sitting in class right now.*
PRESENT PERFECT PROGRESSIVE 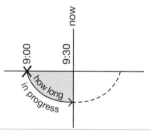	Po is sitting at his desk in class. He sat down at nine o'clock. It is now nine-thirty. (e) Po *has been sitting* in class since nine o'clock. (f) Po *has been sitting* in class for thirty minutes.	The present perfect progressive *emphasizes the duration* (length of time) of an activity that began in the past and is in progress right now. *INCORRECT: Po is sitting in class since nine o'clock.*

(g) CORRECT: I *know* Yoko. (h) INCORRECT: I *am knowing* Yoko. (i) CORRECT: I *have known* Yoko for two years. (j) INCORRECT: I *have been knowing* Yoko for two years.	NOTE: Non-action verbs (e.g., *know, like, own, belong*) are generally not used in the progressive tenses.* In (i): With non-action verbs, the present perfect is used with **since** or **for** to express the duration of a situation that began in the past and continues to the present.

*See Chart 1-6, Verbs Not Usually Used in the Progressive, p. 18.

EXERCISE 31 ▸ Looking at grammar. (Chart 4-6)

Complete the sentences. Use the present progressive or the present perfect progressive form of the verbs in parentheses.

At School

1. I (*sit*) _____am sitting_____ in the cafeteria right now. I (*sit*) _____have been sitting_____ here since twelve o'clock.

2. Kate is standing in line at the registration counter. She (*wait*) _____ for help. She (*wait*) _____ for help for twenty minutes.

3. Scott and Rebecca (*study*) _____ together right now. They (*study*) _____ together in the library for over an hour.

4. Right now we're in class. We (*do*) _____ an exercise. We (*do*) _____ this exercise for a couple of minutes.

5. A: You look busy right now. What (*you, do*) _____?

   B: I (*work*) _____ on my physics experiment. It's a difficult experiment.

   A: How long (*you, work*) _____ on it?

   B: I started planning it last January. I (*work*) _____ on it since then.

EXERCISE 32 ▸ Let's talk. (Chart 4-6)

Answer the questions your teacher asks. Your book is closed.

Example:

TEACHER: Where are you living?
STUDENT: I'm living in an apartment on Fourth Avenue.
TEACHER: How long have you been living there?
STUDENT: I've been living there since last September.

1. Right now you are sitting in class. How long have you been sitting here?
2. When did you first begin to study English? How long have you been studying English?
3. I began to teach English in (*year*). How long have I been teaching English?
4. I began to work at this school in (*month or year*). How long have I been working here?
5. What are we doing right now? How long have we been doing it?
6. (*Student's name*), I see that you wear glasses. How long have you been wearing glasses?
7. Who drives? When did you first drive a car? How long have you been driving?
8. Who drinks coffee? How old were you when you started to drink coffee? How long have you been drinking coffee?
9. Who owns a motorcycle? How long have you owned one?
10. Who likes candy? How long have you liked candy?

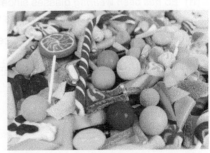

EXERCISE 33 ▸ Warm-up. (Chart 4-7)

Read the sentences and answer this question: *Who is Suzanne helping right now?*

1. Roger is having trouble with math. Suzanne has been helping him with his homework tonight. She has been helping him since 6:00.

2. Suzanne likes to help students with math. She has helped Tia and Kofi this week.

4-7	Present Perfect Progressive vs. Present Perfect

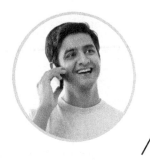 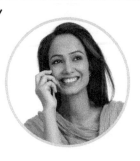

Present Perfect Progressive

(a) Tarik and Gina are talking on the phone. They *have been talking* on the phone for 20 minutes.	The present perfect progressive expresses the *duration of present activities,* using action verbs, as in (a). The activity began in the past and is still in progress.

Present Perfect

(b) Tarik *has talked* to Gina on the phone many times (before now). (c) INCORRECT: *Tarik has been talking to Gina on the phone many times.* (d) Tarik *has known* Gina for two years. (e) INCORRECT: *Tarik has been knowing Gina for two years.*	The present perfect expresses (1) repeated activities that occur at *unspecified times in the past,* as in (b), OR (2) the *duration of present situations,* as in (d), using non-action verbs.

Present Perfect Progressive and Present Perfect

(f) I *have been living* here for six months. OR (g) I *have lived* here for six months. (h) Ed *has been wearing* glasses since he was ten. OR Ed *has worn* glasses since he was ten. (i) I've *been going* to school ever since I was five years old. OR I've *gone* to school ever since I was five years old.	For some (not all) verbs, duration can be expressed by either the present perfect or the present perfect progressive. Examples (f) and (g) have essentially the same meaning, and both are correct. Often either tense can be used with verbs that express the *duration of usual or habitual activities/ situations* (things that happen daily or regularly). Common verbs are *live, work, study, play, teach,* and *wear glasses.*

EXERCISE 34 ▶ Looking at grammar. (Chart 4-7)

Complete the sentences with the verbs in *italics*. Use the present perfect progressive form for the activity that is still in progress.

1. *has been helping / has helped*

   a. Professor Ruiz got to his office at 7:00 A.M. He _____ a student since then.

   b. Professor Jackson is really nice. He _____ me several times with my medical school application.

2. *has been sleeping / has slept*

   a. Tony _____ this afternoon. He stayed up all night to study for a test.

   b. Gina got a new mattress for her dorm room. She _____ on it twice, but it's too hard for her.

3. *have been reading / have read*

   a. I _____ this same page in my chemistry book three times, and I still don't understand it.

   b. I _____ it for the last half hour. It's like another language!

EXERCISE 35 ▶ Looking at grammar. (Chapters 1, 2, and 4)

Look at each set of sentences. Check (✓) the sentences that are still in progress. Look at the verbs in green, and discuss the differences in meaning.

1. a. _____ Rachel is taking English classes.
   b. _____ Nadia has been taking English classes for two months.

2. a. _____ Ayako has been living in Jerusalem for two years. She likes it there.
   b. _____ Beatriz has lived in Jerusalem. She's also lived in Paris. She's lived in New York and Tokyo. She's lived in lots of cities.

3. a. _____ Jack has visited his aunt and uncle many times.
   b. _____ Matt has been visiting his aunt and uncle for the last three days.

4. a. _____ Cyril is talking on the phone.
   b. _____ Cyril talks on the phone a lot.
   c. _____ Cyril has been talking to his boss on the phone for half an hour.
   d. _____ Cyril has talked to his boss on the phone lots of times.

5. a. _____ Mr. Woods walks his dog in Forest Park every day.
   b. _____ Mr. Woods has walked his dog in Forest Park many times.
   c. _____ Mr. Woods walked his dog in Forest Park five times last week.
   d. _____ Mr. Woods is walking his dog in Forest Park right now.
   e. _____ Mr. Woods has been walking his dog in Forest Park since two o'clock.

EXERCISE 36 ▸ Looking at grammar. (Chapter 1 and Charts 4-1 → 4-7)
Choose the correct verb. In some sentences, more than one answer may be possible.

Frustrations

1. I _____ the windows twice, and they still don't look clean.
   a. am washing   b. have washed   c. have been washing

2. Please tell Mira to get off the phone. She _____ for over an hour.
   a. is talking   b. has talked   c. has been talking

3. Where are you? I _____ at the mall for you to pick me up.
   a. wait   b. am waiting   c. have been waiting

4. Josh _____ up all night twice this week. He has a lot of homework.
   a. stays   b. has stayed   c. has been staying

5. Where have you been? The baby _____, and I can't comfort her.
   a. cries   b. is crying   c. has been crying

EXERCISE 37 ▸ Listening. (Chart 4-7)
Listen to the weather report. Then listen again and complete the
sentences with the words you hear.

Do you know these words?
- boy (as an exclamation)
- what's in store
- hail
- weather system
- high winds
- rough

TODAY'S WEATHER

The weather _____ certainly _____ today. Boy, what
a day! _____ already _____ rain, wind, hail, and sun. So,
what's in store for tonight? As you _____ probably _____, dark
clouds _____. We have a weather system moving in that is
going to bring colder temperatures and high winds. _____
all week that this system is coming, and it looks like tonight is it! _____ even
_____ snow down south of us, and we could get some snow here too. So
hang onto your hats! We may have a rough night ahead of us.

EXERCISE 38 ▶ Looking at grammar. (Chart 4-7)

Complete the sentences. Use the present perfect or the present perfect progressive form of the verbs in parentheses. In some sentences, either form is possible.

Enjoying the Outdoors

1. A: I'd like to take a break. We (*hike*) _____*have been hiking*_____ for more than an hour.

   B: OK, let's stop here. The views are beautiful.

2. A: Is the trail to Glacier Lake difficult?

   B: No, not at all. I (*hike*) _____*have hiked*_____ it many times with my kids.

3. A: Do you like it here?

   B: I love it! I (*live*) _*have been living / have lived*_ here since the beginning of the summer

   and (*take*) _____ several beautiful hikes.

4. A: I'm getting hungry. We (*walk*) _____ since sunrise.

   I think I'll have lunch.

   B: Good idea.

5. A: Do you like this campsite?

   B: Very much. I (*stay*) _____ here several times. It's my favorite place

   to camp.

6. A: It's snowing. It (*snow*) _____ all night.

   B: The skiing will be great!

7. A: Do you ski often?

   B: Every day! I (*work*) _____ as a ski instructor here for the past

   five months.

   A: (*you, teach*) _____ for a long time?

   B: I (*teach*) _____ people to ski since I was a teenager.

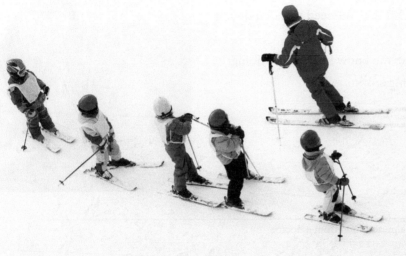
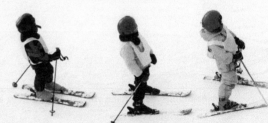

EXERCISE 39 ▸ Listening. (Charts 4-3 → 4-7)
Listen to each conversation and choose the sentence that best describes it.

Example: You will hear: A: This movie is silly.
B: I agree. It's really dumb.

You will choose: (a.) The couple has been watching a movie.
b. The couple finished watching a movie.

1. a. The speakers listened to the radio already.
   b. The speakers have been listening to the radio.

2. a. The man lived in Dubai a year ago.
   b. The man still lives in Dubai.

3. a. The man has called the children several times.
   b. The man called the children once.

4. a. The speakers went to a party and are still there.
   b. The speakers went to a party and have already left.

EXERCISE 40 ▸ Listening and speaking. (Chapters 1 → 4)
Part I. Listen to the phone conversation between a mother and her daughter, Lara.

A Common Illness

LARA: Hi, Mom. I was just calling to tell you that I can't come to your birthday party this weekend. I'm afraid I'm sick.

MOM: Oh, I'm sorry to hear that.

LARA: Yeah, I got sick Wednesday night, and it's just been getting worse.

MOM: Are you going to see a doctor?

LARA: I don't know. I don't want to go to a doctor if it's not serious.

MOM: Well, what symptoms have you been having?

LARA: I've had a cough, and now I have a fever.

MOM: Have you been taking any medicine?

LARA: Just over-the-counter* stuff.

MOM: If your fever doesn't go away, I think you need to call a doctor.

LARA: Yeah, I probably will.

MOM: Well, call me tomorrow, and let me know how you're doing.

LARA: OK. I'll call you in the morning.

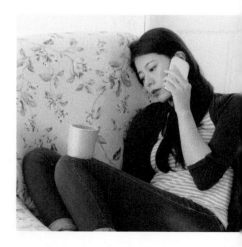

*over-the-counter = medicine you can buy without a prescription from a doctor

Part II. Work with a partner. Complete the conversation and practice it. Take turns being the parent and the sick person.

> *Possible symptoms:*
>
> | | | | | |
> |---|---|---|---|---|
> | a fever | chills | a sore throat | a runny nose | achiness |
> | a stomachache | a cough | a headache | sneezing | nausea |

A: Hi, Mom/Dad. I was just calling to tell you that I can't come to _____. I'm afraid I'm sick.

B: Oh, I'm sorry to hear that.

A: Yeah, I got sick Wednesday night, and it's just been getting worse.

B: Are you going to see a doctor?

A: I don't know. I don't want to go to a doctor if it's not serious.

B: Well, what symptoms have you been having?

A: I've had _____, and now I have _____.

B: Have you been taking any medicine?

A: Just over-the-counter stuff.

B: If your _____ doesn't go away, I think you need to call a doctor.

A: Yeah, I probably will.

B: Well, call me tomorrow and let me know how you're doing.

A: OK. I'll call you in the morning.

EXERCISE 41 ▸ Warm-up. (Charts 4-8)

Read Karen's statement. Which sentence (a. or b.) is correct?

> KAREN: Jay met me for lunch. He was so happy. He had passed his driver's test.
> a. First, Jay talked to Karen. Then he passed his test.
> b. First, Jay passed his test. Then he talked to Karen.

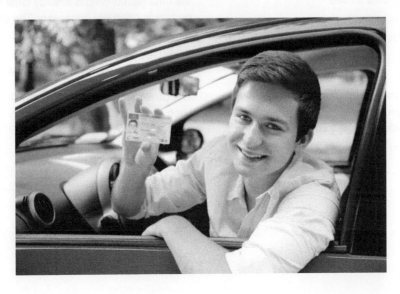

Situation:
Jack left his office at 2:00. Mia arrived at his office at 2:15 and knocked on the door.

(a) When Mia arrived, Jack wasn't there. He *had left*.

(b) *By the time* Mia arrived, Jack *had already left*.

The PAST PERFECT is used when the speaker is talking about two different events at two different times in the past; one event ended before the second event happened.

In (a): There are two events, and both happened in the past: *Jack left his office. Mia arrived at his office.*

To show the time relationship between the two events, we use the past perfect (***had left***) to say that the first event (Jack leaving his office) was completed before the second event (Mia arriving at his office) occurred.

In (b): ***By the time*** is frequently used with the past perfect to indicate one event happened before another.

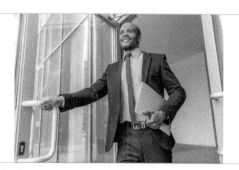

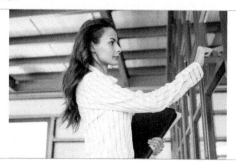

(c) Jack *had left* his office when Mia arrived.	FORM: ***had*** + *past participle*
(d) He*'d* left. I*'d* left. They*'d* left. Etc.	CONTRACTION: *I / you / she / he / it / we / they* + ***'d***

(e) Jack *had left* before Mia arrived. (f) Jack *left* before Mia arrived. (g) Mia *arrived* after Jack had left. (h) Mia *arrived* after Jack left.	When ***before*** and ***after*** are used in a sentence, the time relationship is already clear so the past perfect is often not necessary. The simple past may be used, as in (f) and (h). Examples (e) and (f) have the same meaning. Examples (g) and (h) have the same meaning.

(i) Stella was alone in a strange city. She walked down the avenue slowly, looking in shop windows. Suddenly, she turned her head and looked behind her. Someone *had called* her name.	The past perfect is more common in formal writing such as fiction, as in (i).

EXERCISE 42 ▸ Looking at grammar. (Chart 4-8)
Identify which action in the past took place first (1st) and which action took place second (2nd).

1. Before I went to bed, I checked the front door. My roommate had already locked it.
   a. ___2nd___ I checked the door.
   b. ___1st___ My roommate locked the door.

2. I looked for Diego, but he had left the building.
   a. _____ Diego left the building.
   b. _____ I looked for Diego.

3. I laughed when I saw my son. He had poured a bowl of noodles on top of his head.
   a. _____ I laughed.
   b. _____ My son poured a bowl of noodles on his head.

4. Oliver arrived at the theater on time, but he couldn't get in. He had left his ticket at home.
   a. _____ Oliver left his ticket at home.
   b. _____ Oliver arrived at the theater.

5. I handed Betsy the newspaper, but she didn't want it. She had read it during her lunch hour.
   a. _____ I handed Betsy the newspaper.
   b. _____ Betsy read the newspaper.

6. After Carl arrived in New York, he called his mother. He had promised to call her as soon as he got in.
   a. _____ Carl made a promise to his mother.
   b. _____ Carl called his mother.

7. The tennis player jumped in the air for joy. He had won the match.
   a. _____ The tennis player won the match.
   b. _____ The tennis player jumped in the air.

EXERCISE 43 ▸ **Looking at grammar.** (Charts 4-3, 4-4, and 4-8)
Complete the conversations with the present perfect or past perfect. Use *have*, *has*, or *had*.

1. A: There's Professor Newton. I'll introduce you.
   B: You don't need to. I _____ already met him.

2. A: Did Jack introduce you to Professor Newton?
   B: He didn't need to. I _____ already met him before I moved here.

3. A: Oh, no! We're too late. The train _____ left.
   B: That's OK. We'll catch the next one.

4. A: Tom missed the train.
   B: I know. I was with him. When we got to the station, the train _____ just left.

5. A: You sure woke up early this morning!
   B: Well, I went to bed early last night. By 6:00 A.M., I _____ already slept for eight hours.

6. A: Go back to sleep. It's only 6:00 in the morning.
   B: I can't. I _____ been awake since 5:00.

7. A: Grandpa _____ gone back into the hospital again.
   B: What happened?
   A: When Grandma got home last night, she found him on the floor. He _____ fallen and hit his head.

EXERCISE 44 ▸ **Check your knowledge.** (Chapter 4 Review)
Correct the errors in verb tense usage.

My Experience with English

           studying
1. I have been s~~tudied~~ English for eight years, but I still have a lot to learn.

2. I start English classes at this school two months ago, and I have learned a lot of English since then.

3. I want to learn English since I am a child.

4. I have been thinking about how to improve my English skills quickly since I came here, but I hadn't found a good way.

5. Our teacher likes to give tests. We has have six tests since the beginning of the term.

6. I like learning English. When I was young, my father found an Australian girl to teach my brothers and me English, but when we move to another city, my father didn't find anyone to teach us.

7. I made many friends since school started. I meet Abdul in the cafeteria on the first day. He was

   friendly and kind. We are friends since that day.

8. Abdul have been study English for three months. His English is better than mine.

EXERCISE 45 ▶ Reading, grammar, and writing. (Chapters 1, 2, and 4)
Part I. Read the passage. <u>Underline</u> the words that express time. Note the verbs in green.

A Brief Introduction

My name is Tanet Sakda. I am from Thailand. <u>Right now</u> I am studying English at this school. I have been at this school since the beginning of January. I arrived here on January 2, and my classes began on January 6.

Since I came here, I have done many things, and I have met many people. Last week, I went to a party at my friend's house. I met some of the other students from Thailand at the party. Of course, we spoke Thai, so I didn't practice my English that night. There were only people from Thailand at the party.

However, since I came here, I have made friends with a lot of other people too, including people from Latin America and the Middle East. I have enjoyed meeting people from other countries, and they have become my friends. Now I know people from around the world.

Part II. Write three paragraphs about yourself. Use Part I as a model. Answer these questions:

Paragraph I:

1. What is your name? _____

2. Where are you from? _____

3. How long have you been here? _____

Paragraph II:

4. What have you done since you came here? OR What have you learned since you began

   studying English? _____

   _____

Paragraph III:

5. Who(m) have you met in this class? OR Who(m) have you met recently?

   _____

   _____

6. Give a little information about these people.

   _____

   _____

WRITING TIP

The English verb system can seem very confusing. Small differences in verb forms can change the meaning of a sentence. A good way to check your writing is to focus on one verb form at a time. For example, choose a time word like *now*. Find all the instances of *now* and check that the verbs are in the correct tense. That is probably present progressive for this writing assignment. Note that sometimes, there is only one time word for several sentences that follow.

Then choose another time word and think about the verb tenses for that time. Check that they are correct.

Later, for a final check, go through your paragraphs sentence by sentence to check your verbs one last time.

Here are some helpful time markers and the tenses they often go with:

Time Markers	Tense(s)
now, today	present progressive
last night / week / etc. *that night / week / etc.* *yesterday* *in 2010* (specific date)	simple past
since, for	present perfect, simple past* OR present perfect progressive (for events still in progress)

*Remember: when you introduce a time clause with *since*, the main clause uses present perfect and the *since*-clause uses the simple past.

Part III. Edit your writing. Check for the following:

1. ☐ use of the simple past for finished events
2. ☐ use of the present perfect for events up to now
3. ☐ use of the present perfect for unspecified time
4. ☐ use of the present perfect progressive for events that started in the past and are still in progress
5. ☐ correct use of **have** and **has** with the present perfect and present perfect progressive
6. ☐ correct spelling (use a dictionary or spell-check)

▪▪▪▪▪ For digital resources, go to the Pearson Practice English app.

PRETEST: What do I already know?

Write "C" if the **boldfaced** words are correct and "I" if they are incorrect.

1. _____ **Has** it snowing right now? (Chart 5-1)

2. _____ **When** will you graduate from college? (Chart 5-2)

3. _____ **What** did you say that **for**? (Chart 5-3)

4. _____ Who(m) **you asked** to the wedding? (Chart 5-4)

5. _____ What **did happen** at the party last night? (Chart 5-3)

6. _____ What is your father's occupation — what **is he do**? (Chart 5-4)

7. _____ **Which websites** do you check most often? (Chart 5-5)

8. _____ **How many years** are you? (Chart 5-6)

9. _____ **How often** do you see your parents? (Chart 5-7)

10. _____ **How far is** from Tokyo to Singapore? (Chart 5-8)

11. _____ **How long it take** to fly from Berlin to Prague? (Chart 5-9)

12. _____ **How do you spell** the word *shampoo*? (Chart 5-11)

13. _____ **How about getting** takeout for dinner tonight? (Chart 5-12)

14. _____ There's enough money for the rent, **isn't it?** (Chart 5-13)

EXERCISE 1 ▶ Warm-up. (Chart 5-1)

Choose the correct completion.

A: _____ you like sweets?

    a. Are   c. Have

    b. Do   d. Were

B: Yes, _____.

    a. I like   c. I have

    b. I'm   d. I do

5-1 Yes/No Questions and Short Answers

Yes/No Question	Short Answer (+ Long Answer)	
(a) *Are you* ready? *Are you* a student?	*Yes, I am.* (I am ready.) *No, I am not.* (I'm not a student.)	A **yes/no** question is a question that can be answered by *yes* or *no*. * In (b): *INCORRECT: Yes, I like.*
(b) *Do you like* tea?	*Yes, I do.* (I like tea.) *No, I don't.* (I don't like tea.)	
(c) *Is it raining?*	*Yes, it is.* (It's raining.) *No, it isn't.* (It isn't raining.)	In an affirmative short answer (*yes*), a helping verb is NOT contracted with the subject.
(d) *Did Liz call?*	*Yes, she did.* (Liz called.) *No, she didn't.* (Liz didn't call.)	
(e) *Have you met* Al?	*Yes, I have.* (I have met Al.) *No, I haven't.* (I haven't met Al.)	In (c): *INCORRECT: Yes, it's.* In (e): *INCORRECT: Yes, I've.* In (f): *INCORRECT: Yes, he'll.*
(f) *Will Rob be* here?	*Yes, he will.* (Rob will be here.) *No, he won't.* (Rob won't be here.)	The spoken emphasis in a short answer is on the verb.
(g) *Is there* a restroom nearby?	**Yes, *there is.*** (There is a restroom nearby.) No, *there isn't.* (There isn't a restroom nearby.)	**Be** + *there* asks if something exists somewhere.

*For more information on question formation with the tenses in this chart, see Charts 1-7, p. 21, 2-1, p. 31, 2-2, p. 32, 3-2, p. 66, 3-3, p. 69, and 4-2, p. 94.

EXERCISE 2 ▸ Looking at grammar. (Chart 5-1)
Choose the correct verbs.

A New Cell Phone

1. A: Is / Does   that your new cell phone?
   B: Yes, it   is / does.

2. A: Are / Do   you like it?
   B: Yes, I   am / do.

3. A: Were / Did   you buy it online?
   B: Yes, I   was / did.

4. A: Was / Did   it expensive?
   B: No, it   wasn't / didn't.

5. A: Is / Does   it ringing right now?
   B: Yes, it   is / does.

6. A: Are / Do   you going to answer it?
   B: Yes, I   am / do.

7. A: Was / Did   the call important?
   B: Yes, it   was / did.

8. A: Have / Were   you turned your phone off?
   B: No, I   haven't / wasn't.

9. A: Will / Are   you call me later?
   B: Yes, I   will / are.

10. A: Do / Are   you have my new number?
    B: Yes, I   do / have.

EXERCISE 3 ▸ Looking at grammar. (Chart 5-1)

Use the information in parentheses to make *yes/no* questions. Complete each conversation with an appropriate short answer. Do not use a negative verb in the question.

Travel Questions

1. A: ___Do you take credit cards?___

   B: Yes, ___we do.___ (We take credit cards.)

2. A: _____

   B: No, _____ (The price doesn't include tax.)

3. A: _____

   B: Yes, _____ (You need a reservation.)

4. A: _____

   B: Yes, _____ (We are open every day.)

5. A: _____

   B: No, _____ (The tour isn't going to leave soon.)

6. A: _____

   B: Yes, _____ (The bus came.)

7. A: _____

   B: No, _____ (You haven't missed the flight.)

8. A: _____

   B: Yes, _____ (There is an express train.)

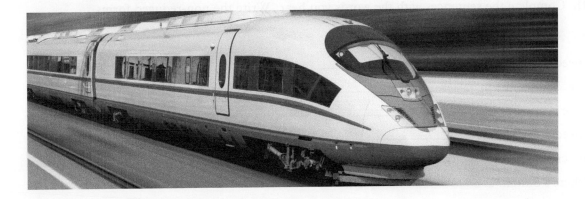

EXERCISE 4 ▸ Let's talk: interview. (Chart 5-1)

Interview seven students in your class. Make questions with the given words. Ask each student a different question.

1. you \ like \ animals?
2. you \ ever \ had \ a pet snake?
3. it \ be \ cold \ in this room?
4. it \ rain \ right now?
5. you \ sleep \ well last night?
6. you \ be \ tired right now?
7. you \ be \ here next year?

EXERCISE 5 ▸ Looking at grammar. (Chart 5-1)

Complete the questions with **Do, Does, Did, Is,** or **Are**.

Leaving for the Airport

1. We're ready to leave. _____ you have your passport?

2. _____ you almost ready?

3. _____ you already print out our boarding passes?

4. _____ you remember to pack a snack for the plane?

5. Your carry-on looks big. _____ it fit under the seat?

6. _____ you call for our ride?

7. _____ our ride coming soon?

8. _____ the driver nearby?

EXERCISE 6 ▸ Listening. (Chart 5-1)

In spoken English, it may be hard to hear the beginning of a *yes/no* question because the words are often reduced.*

Part I. Listen to these common reductions.

1. Is he absent?	→	*Ih-ze* absent? or *Ze* absent?
2. Is she absent?	→	*Ih-she* absent?
3. Does it work?	→	*Zit* work?
4. Did it break?	→	*Dih-dit* break? or *Dit* break?
5. Has he been sick?	→	*Ze* been sick? or *A-ze* been sick?
6. Is there enough?	→	*Zere* enough?
7. Is that OK?	→	*Zat* OK?

Part II. Complete the sentences with the words you hear. Write the non-reduced forms.

At the Grocery Store

1. I need to see the manager. _____ available?

2. I need to see the manager. _____ in the store today?

3. Here is one bag of apples. _____ enough?

4. I need a drink of water. _____ a drinking fountain?

5. My credit card isn't working. Hmmm. _____ expire?

6. Where's Simon? _____ left?

7. The price seems high. _____ include the tax?

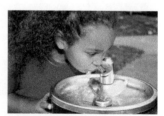

a drinking fountain

---

*See also Chapter 1, Exercise 37, p. 24, and Chapter 2, Exercise 19, p. 41.

EXERCISE 7 ▸ Warm-up. (Chart 5-2)

Choose the correct answers. There may be more than one answer for each question.

1. Where did you go?
   a. To the hospital.   b. Yes, I did.   c. Outside.   d. Yesterday.

2. When is James leaving?
   a. I'm not sure.   b. Yes, he is.   c. Yes, he does.   d. Around noon.

3. Why did Mr. and Ms. Lee move?
   a. I think so.   b. They got new jobs.   c. No, they aren't.   d. Yes, they did.

5-2 Where, Why, When, What Time, How Come, What ... For

The questions in this chart ask for information. Note that most are *wh*-type questions. The answers do not begin with *yes* or *no*.*

Question	Answer	
(a) *Where* did he go?	Home.	*Where* asks about *place*.
(b) *When* did he leave?	Last night. Two days ago. Monday morning. Seven-thirty.	A question with *when* can be answered by any time expression, as in the sample answers in (b).
(c) *What time* did he leave?	Seven-thirty. Around five o'clock. A quarter past ten.	A question with *what time* asks about *time on a clock*.
(d) *Why* did he leave?	Because he didn't feel well.**	*Why* asks about *reason*.
(e) *What* did he leave *for*? (f) *How come* he left?	*Why* can also be expressed with the phrases *What ... for* and *How come*, as in (e) and (f). Note that with *How come,* usual question order is not used. The subject precedes the verb and no form of *do* is used.	

*For a comparison of *yes/no* and information questions, see Appendix A-8.

**See Chart 8-6, p. 241, for the use of *because*. *Because I didn't feel well* is an adverb clause. It is not a complete sentence. In this example, it is the short answer to a question.

EXERCISE 8 ▸ Reading and grammar. (Charts 5-1 and 5-2)

Read the information about Irina and Paul. Then make complete questions with the given words. Choose the correct short answers.

The Simple Life

Irina and Paul live a simple life. They have a one-room cabin on a mountain lake. They fish for some of their food. They also raise chickens. They pick fruit from trees and berries from bushes in the summer. They don't have electricity or TV, but they enjoy their life. They don't need a lot to be happy.

1. QUESTION: where \ Irina and Paul \ live?
   Where do Irina and Paul live?
   ANSWER: a. Yes, they do.   (b.) On a lake.

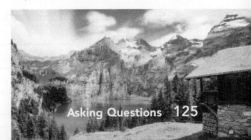

2. QUESTION: they \ live \ a simple life? _____

   ANSWER: a. Yes, they live.   b. Yes, they do.

3. QUESTION: when \ they \ pick \ fruit from trees? _____

   ANSWER: a. In the summer.   b. Yes, they do.

4. QUESTION: they \ have \ electricity? _____

   ANSWER: a. No, they don't.   b. No, they don't have.

5. QUESTION: they \ enjoy \ their life? _____

   ANSWER: a. Yes, they do.   b. Yes, they enjoy.

6. QUESTION: they \ be \ happy? _____

   ANSWER: a. Yes, they do.   b. Yes, they are.

EXERCISE 9 ▸ Looking at grammar. (Chart 5-2)

Restate the sentences with **How come** and **What for**.

1. Why are you going?   3. Why does he need more money?
2. Why did they come?   4. Why are they going to leave?

EXERCISE 10 ▸ Looking at grammar. (Chart 5-2)

Complete the questions using the information from Speaker A.

What was that?

1. A: I'm going downtown in a few minutes.

   B: I didn't catch that. When ___are you going downtown___? OR

   B: I didn't catch that. Where ___are you going in a few minutes___?

2. A: My kids are transferring to Lakeview Elementary School because it's a better school.

   B: What was that? Where _____? OR

   B: What was that? Why _____?

3. A: I am going to meet Taka at 10:00 at the mall.

   B: I couldn't hear you. Tell me again. What time _____? OR

   B: I couldn't hear you. Tell me again. Where _____?

4. A: Class begins at 8:15.

   B: Are you sure? When _____? OR

   B: Are you sure? What time _____?

5. A: I stayed home from work because I wanted to watch the World Cup final on TV.

   B: Huh?! Why _____? OR

   B: Huh?! What _____ for?

EXERCISE 11 ▶ Grammar and listening. (Charts 5-1 and 5-2)
Complete the conversation. Then listen to the conversation to check your answers. Use a form of
be going to for the future verb.

Where are Roberto and Isabelle?

A: _Do you know_ ___1___ Roberto and Isabelle?

B: Yes, I ___2___. They live around the corner from me.

A: ___3___ seen them recently?

B: No, I ___4___. They're out of town.

A: When ___5___ be back? I'm having a party, and I can't

reach them.

B: They're going to be back Monday. They

are with Roberto's parents.

A: Oh, ___6___ they there?

B: Because his dad is sick.

A: That's too bad.

B: ___7___ want Roberto's or

Isabelle's cell number?

A: No, I don't, but thanks. I'll talk to them when they get back.

B: OK, sounds good.

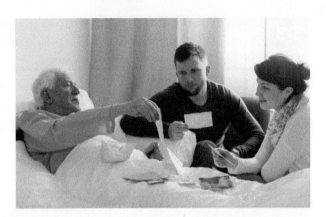

 EXERCISE 12 ▶ Listening. (Charts 5-1 and 5-2)
Listen to each question and choose the correct answer.

Example: You will hear: When are you leaving?
You will choose: a. Yes, I am. (b.) Tomorrow. c. In the city.

1. a. I am too. b. Yesterday. c. Sure.

2. a. For dinner. b. At 6:00. c. At the restaurant.

3. a. Outside the mall. b. After lunch. c. Because I need a ride.

4. a. At work. b. Because traffic was heavy. c. A few hours ago.

5. a. The kitchen. b. In a few minutes. c. My parents are coming.

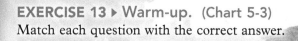

EXERCISE 13 ▸ Warm-up. (Chart 5-3)
Match each question with the correct answer.

A Flight to Rome

1. Who flew to Rome? _____
2. Who did you fly to Rome? _____
3. What did you fly to Rome? _____
4. What flew to Rome? _____

a. A small plane flew to Rome.
b. I flew to Rome.
c. I flew a small plane to Rome.
d. I flew Pablo to Rome.

5-3 Questions With *Who, Whom,* and *What*

Question	Answer	

(a) ^S *Who* came?	^S *Someone* came.	In (a): **Who** is used as the subject (S) of a question.
		
		In (b): **Who(m)** is used as the object (O) in a question.
		
		Whom is used in formal written and spoken English. In everyday English, **who** is usually used instead of **whom**:
		  UNCOMMON: Whom did you see?
		  COMMON: Who did you see?

(b) ^O *Who(m)* did *you* see?	^S *I* saw ^O *someone.*	

(c) ^S *What* happened?	^S *Something* happened.	**What** can be used as either the subject or the object in a question.
		
		Note in (a) and (c): When **who** or **what** is used as the subject of a question, usual question word order is not used; no form of **do** is used:
		  CORRECT: Who came?
		  INCORRECT: Who did come?

(d) ^O *What* did *you* see?	^S *I* saw ^O *something.*	

EXERCISE 14 ▸ Looking at grammar. (Chart 5-3)
Make questions with **Who, Who(m)**, and **What**. Write "S" if the question word is the subject.
Write "O" if the question word is the object.

What's going on?

	QUESTION	ANSWER
1.	*^S Who knows?*	^S *Someone* knows.
2.	*^O Who(m) did you see?*	^O I saw *someone.*
3.	_____	*Someone* is outside.

4. _____   Talya met someone.

5. _____   Mike found out something.

6. _____   Something changed Gina's mind.

7. _____   Gina is talking about someone.*

8. _____   Gina is talking about something.

EXERCISE 15 ▸ Looking at grammar. (Chart 5-3)
Complete the questions with **Who** or **What**.

At the Hospital

1. A: _____ just left?

   B: That was the doctor.

2. A: _____ do you need?

   B: A glass of water.

3. A: _____ is your nurse today?

   B: I'm not sure. Maybe David or Nancy.

4. A: _____ is going on?

   B: I'm getting a new roommate.

5. A: _____ did you call?

   B: The nurse.

6. A: _____ do you need?

   B: Dr. Smith or her nurse.

EXERCISE 16 ▸ Let's talk. (Chart 5-3)
Abbreviations in text messages are very popular. Ask your classmates the meaning of these abbreviations.

Example: LOL
STUDENT A: What does *LOL* mean?
STUDENT B: *LOL* means "laughing out loud."

1. TTYL   5. IMHO   8. XOXO
2. BTW   6. TYT   9. OMW
3. ROTFL   7. ILY   10. GTG
4. IMO

---

*A preposition may come at the beginning of a question in very formal English:
   About whom (NOT *who*) is *Tina talking?*
In everyday English, a preposition usually does not come at the beginning of a question.

EXERCISE 17 ▸ Let's talk: interview. (Chart 5-3)
Walk around the room and ask your classmates questions with **Who** or **What**.

Example: _____ are you currently reading?
STUDENT A: What are you currently reading?
STUDENT B: A book about a cowboy.

1. _____ do you like to do in your free time?

2. _____ is your idea of the perfect vacation?

3. _____ is your best friend?

4. _____ was an important teacher from your childhood?

5. _____ stresses you out?

6. _____ do you need that you don't have?

7. _____ would you most like to invite to dinner? Why? (*The person can be living or dead.*)

EXERCISE 18 ▸ Listening. (Charts 5-2 and 5-3)
Listen to the conversation. Listen again and complete
the sentences with the words you hear.

A Secret

A: John told me something.

B: _____ tell you?
     1

A: It's confidential. I can't tell you.

B: _____ anyone else?
     2

A: He told a few other people.

B: _____ tell?
     3

A: Some friends.

B: Then it's not a secret. _____ say?
                                  4

A: I can't tell you.

B: _____ can't _____ me?
     5   6

A: Because it's about you. But don't worry. It's nothing bad.

B: Gee. Thanks a lot. That sure makes me feel better.

EXERCISE 19 ▸ Reading, grammar, and speaking. (Charts 5-2 and 5-3)
Read the passage about Nina's birthday. Make questions with the given words. Answer the
questions with a partner, in small groups, or as a class.

The Birthday Present

Tom got home late last night, around midnight. His wife, Nina, was sitting on the couch waiting for him. She was quite worried because Tom is never late.

Tomorrow is Nina's birthday. Unfortunately, Tom doesn't think she will be happy with her birthday present. Yesterday, Tom bought her a bike, and he decided to ride it home from the bike shop. While he was riding down a hill, a driver came too close to him, and he landed in a ditch. Tom was OK, but the bike wasn't. Tom walked to a bus stop nearby and finally got home.

Tom told Nina the story, but Nina didn't care about the bike. She said she had a better present: her husband.

> Do you know these words?
> - couch   - landed
> - quite   - ditch

1. When \ Tom \ get home
2. Where \ be \ his wife
3. What \ Tom \ buy
4. Why \ be \ Tom \ late
5. What present \ Nina \ get

EXERCISE 20 ▸ Warm-up. (Chart 5-4)

Answer the questions with information about yourself.

1. What do you do on weekends? I ...
2. What did you do last weekend? I ...
3. What are you going to do this weekend? I'm going to ...
4. What will you do the following weekend? I will ...

5-4 Using *What* + a Form of *Do*

Question	Answer	
(a) *What **does** Bob **do** every morning?*	He *goes to class.*	***What** + a form of **do*** is used to ask questions about activities.
(b) *What **did** you **do** yesterday?*	I *went downtown.*	Examples of forms of ***do***: *am doing, will do, are going to do, did, etc.*
(c) *What **is** Anna **doing** (right now)?*	She's *studying.*	
(d) *What **are** you **going to do** tomorrow?*	I'm *going to go to the beach.*	In (g): *What do you do?* has a special meaning. It means *What is your occupation, your job?* Another way of asking the same question: *What do you do for a living?*
(e) *What **do** you **want to do** tonight?*	I *want to go to a movie.*	
(f) *What **would** you **like to do** tomorrow?*	I *would like to visit Jim.*	
(g) *What **do** you **do**?*	I'm *a software engineer.*	

EXERCISE 21 ▸ Looking at grammar. (Chart 5-4)

Make questions beginning with ***What*** + a form of ***do***.

1. A: _____*What are you doing*_____ right now?
   B: I'm working on a monthly budget.

2. A: _____ last night?
   B: I paid my bills.

3. A: _____ tomorrow?

   B: I'm going to go run a lot of errands.

4. A: _____ tomorrow?

   B: I want to go to the beach.

5. A: _____ this evening?

   B: I would like to go to a movie.

6. A: _____ in your business classes?

   B: We do a lot of project work in small groups.

7. A: _____ for your next vacation?

   B: I'm staying home and relaxing. My wife has to work.

8. A: _____ (for a living)?

   B: My wife is a teacher. She teaches first grade.

EXERCISE 22 ▸ Let's talk: interview. (Chart 5-4)
Interview your classmates. Make questions with the given words and **What** + a form of **do**. More than one verb tense may be possible. Share a few of your classmates' answers with the class.

Example: tomorrow
STUDENT A: What are you going to do tomorrow? / What do you want to do tomorrow? / What would you like to do tomorrow? / Etc.
STUDENT B: I'm going to buy a new video game. / I want to buy a new video game. / I'd like to buy a new video game. / Etc.

1. last night	6. last weekend
2. right now	7. after class yesterday
3. next Saturday	8. every morning
4. this afternoon	9. since you arrived in this city
5. tonight	10. on weekends

EXERCISE 23 ▸ Warm-up. (Chart 5-5)
Answer the questions about ice cream. Use the flavors in the box or your own words.

blackberry	chocolate	coffee	lemon	strawberry
caramel	coconut	green tea	mint	vanilla

1. Which ice-cream flavors are popular in your country?
2. What kind of ice cream do you like?

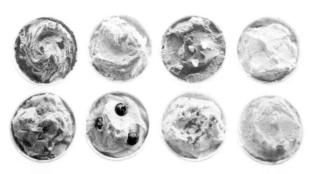

5-5 *Which* vs. *What* and *What Kind Of*

Which

(a) JOE: May I borrow a pen from you? MIA: Sure. I have two pens. This pen has black ink. That pen has red ink. *Which pen* do you want? OR *Which one* do you want? OR *Which* do you want?	In (a): Mia uses *which* (not *what*) because she wants Joe to choose. *Which* is used when the speaker wants someone to make a choice, when the speaker is offering alternatives: *this one or that one; these or those.*
(b) AMY: I like these earrings, and I like those too. ZAC: *Which (earrings / ones)* are you going to buy? AMY: I think I'll get these.	*Which* can be used with either singular or plural nouns.
(c) LEO: Here's a photo of my daughter's class. TIA: Very nice. *Which one* is your daughter?	*Which* can be used to ask about people as well as things.
(d) JAN: My aunt gave me some money for my birthday. I'm going to take it with me to the mall. MAX: *What* are you going to buy with it? JAN: I haven't decided yet.	In (d): The question doesn't involve choosing from a particular group of items, so Max uses *what*, not *which*.

What Kind Of

QUESTION	ANSWER	
		What kind of asks for information about a specific type (a specific kind) in a general category.

(e) *What kind of shoes* did you buy?	Boots.
	Sandals.
	Tennis shoes.
	Loafers.
	Running shoes.
	High heels.
	Clogs.
	Etc.
		In (e): general category = shoes
		  specific kinds = boots
		       sandals
		       tennis shoes
		       etc.

(f) *What kind of fruit* do you like best?	Apples.
	Bananas.
	Oranges.
	Grapefruit.
	Strawberries.
	Etc.
		In (f): general category = fruit
		  specific kinds = apples
		       bananas
		       oranges
		       etc.

EXERCISE 24 ▶ Looking at grammar. (Chart 5-5)
Make questions beginning with **Which** or **What**.

1. A: I have two books. *Which book / Which one / Which do you want?*

   B: That one. (I want that book.)

2. A: *What did you buy when you went shopping?*

   B: A book. (I bought a book when I went shopping.)

3. A: Could I borrow your pen for a minute?

   B: Sure. I have two. _____

   A: That one. (I would like that one.)

4. A: _____

   B: A pen. (Hassan borrowed a pen from me.)

5. A: _____

   B: Two pieces of hard candy. (I have two pieces of hard candy in my hand.) Would you like one?

   A: Yes. Thanks.

   B: _____

   A: The yellow one. (I'd like the yellow one.)

6. A: _____ the most in South America?

   B: Peru and Brazil. (I enjoyed Peru and Brazil the most.) I have family there.

EXERCISE 25 ▶ Let's talk: interview. (Chart 5-5)
Complete the questions with an appropriate word in the box. Then interview classmates.
Write their answers and share some with the class.

animals	electronics	movies	podcasts	social media
desserts	ice cream	music	school subjects	TV shows

1. What kind of _____ do you like to listen to?

   STUDENT 1: _____

   STUDENT 2: _____

2. What kind of _____ do you like to watch?

   STUDENT 1: _____

   STUDENT 2: _____

3. What kind of _____ do you like to eat?

   STUDENT 1: _____

   STUDENT 2: _____

4. What kind of _____ do you use the most?

   STUDENT 1: _____

   STUDENT 2: _____

5. What kind of _____ do you know a lot about?

   STUDENT 1: _____

   STUDENT 2: _____

EXERCISE 26 ▸ Warm-up. (Chart 5-6)
Match each question with the correct answer.

1. How tall is your sister? _____   a. By bus.
2. How old is your brother? _____   b. In five minutes.
3. How did you get here? _____   c. I don't know him at all. I only know his sister.
4. How soon do we need to go? _____   d. Fifteen.
5. How well do you know Kazu? _____   e. Five feet (1.52 meters).

5-6 Using *How*

Question	Answer	
(a) *How* did you get here?	I drove. / By car. I took a taxi. / By taxi. I took a bus. / By bus. I flew. / By plane. I took a train. / By train. I walked. / On foot.	*How* has many uses. One use of *how* is to ask about means (ways) of transportation.
(b) *How old* are you?	Twenty-one.	*How* is often used with adjectives (e.g., *old, big*) and adverbs (e.g., *well, quickly*).
(c) *How tall* is he?	About six feet (1.83 meters).	
(d) *How big* is your apartment?	It has three rooms.	
(e) *How sleepy* are you?	Very sleepy.	
(f) *How hungry* are you?	I'm starving.	
(g) *How soon* will you be ready?	In five minutes.	
(h) *How well* does he speak English?	Very well.	
(i) *How quickly* can you get here?	I can get there in 30 minutes.	

EXERCISE 27 ▸ Reading and grammar. (Chart 5-6)
Read the passage about John and then answer the questions.

Long John

John is 14 years old. He is very tall for his age. He is 6 foot, 6 inches (2 meters). His friends call him "Long John." People are surprised to find out that he is still a teenager. Both his parents are average height, so John's height seems unusual.

It causes problems for him, especially when he travels. Beds in hotels are too short, and there is never enough leg room on airplanes. He is very uncomfortable. When he can, he prefers to take a train because he can walk around and stretch his legs. But John has an advantage over his friends. He's already a great basketball player.

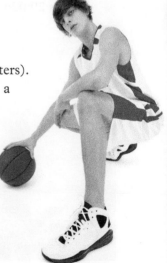

1. How tall is John? _____ .

2. How old is John? _____ .

3. How well do you think he sleeps in hotels? _____ .

4. How comfortable is he on airplanes? _____ .

5. How does he like to travel? _____ .

EXERCISE 28 ▸ Looking at grammar. (Chart 5-6)
Make questions with **How**.

1. A: _How old is your daughter?_ _____
   B: Ten. (My daughter is ten years old.)

2. A: _____
   B: Very important. (Education is very important.)

3. A: _____
   B: By bus. (I get to school by bus.)

4. A: _____
   B: Very, very deep. (The ocean is very, very deep.)

5. A: _____
   B: By plane. (I'm going to get to Buenos Aires by plane.)

6. A: _____
   B: Not very. (The test wasn't very difficult.)

7. A: _____
   B: I ran. (I ran here.)

8. A: _____
   B: In an hour. (We are going to get there in an hour.)

9. A: _____
   B: On foot. (I'll walk to your house.)

10. A: _____
    B: It's 29,029 feet high. (Mount Everest is 29,029 feet high.)*

*29,029 feet = 8,848 meters

Complete the conversations with the words you hear.

1. A: _____ are these eggs?
   B: I just bought them at the farmers' market, so they should be fine.

2. A: _____ were the tickets?
   B: They were 50% off.

3. A: _____ was the driver's test?
   B: Well, I didn't pass, so that gives you an idea.

4. A: _____ is the car?
   B: There's dirt on the floor. We need to vacuum it inside.

5. A: _____ is the frying pan?
   B: Don't touch it! You'll burn yourself.

6. A: _____ is the street you live on?
   B: There is a lot of traffic, so we keep the windows closed a lot.

7. A: _____ are you about interviewing for the job?
   B: Very. I already scheduled an interview with the company.

💬 **EXERCISE 30 ▸ Let's talk: pairwork.** (Charts 5-1 → 5-6)
Work with a partner. Create a conversation between a parent and teenager. You can write any questions that make sense. Practice your conversation, and present it to the class. You can look at your book before you speak. When you speak, look at your partner.

Parent to Teen

A: _____?

B: We're not sure. Maybe we'll go to a movie.

A: _____?

B: My friends.

A: _____?

B: Not too late. Probably around 11:00.

A: _____?

B: We'll take the subway.

A: _____?

B: Because you're asking me so many questions!

A: That's my job. I'm your parent!

EXERCISE 31 ▶ Warm-up: trivia. (Chart 5-7)
Match each question with the best answer.*

1. How often does the earth go completely around the sun? _____

2. How often do the summer Olympics occur? _____

3. How often do earthquakes occur? _____

4. How many times a year can a healthy person safely donate blood? _____

5. How many times a day do the hour and minute hands on a clock overlap? _____

a. About six times a year.

b. Several hundred times a day.

c. Once a year.

d. Every four years.

e. Exactly 22 times a day.

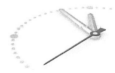

5-7 Using *How Often / How Many Times*

Question	Answer	
(a) *How often* do you go shopping?	Every day. Once a week. About twice a week. Every other day or so.* Three times a month.	*How often* asks about frequency.
(b) *How many times a day* do you eat?	Three or four.	Other ways of asking *how often*:
How many times a week do you go shopping?	Two.	
How many times a month do you go to the post office?	Once.	*how many times* { a day / a week / a month / a year
How many times a year do you take a vacation?	Once or twice.	

Frequency Expressions

a lot	every	
occasionally	every other	
once in a while	once a	day / week / month / year
not very often	twice a	
hardly ever	three times a	
almost never	ten times a	
never		

Every other day means "Monday yes, Tuesday no, Wednesday yes, Thursday no," etc. *Or so* means "approximately."

---

*See *Trivia Answers*, p. 247.

EXERCISE 32 ▸ Let's talk: pairwork. (Chart 5-7)
Work with a partner. Take turns asking and answering questions with **How often** or **How many times a day/week/month/year**.

Example: eat lunch at the cafeteria
PARTNER A: How often/many times a week do you eat lunch at the cafeteria?
PARTNER B: About twice a week. How about you? How often do you eat at the cafeteria?
PARTNER A: I don't. I bring my own lunch.

1. check email
2. listen to podcasts
3. go out to eat
4. cook your own dinner
5. buy a toothbrush
6. take selfies
7. attend weddings
8. stream music from the internet

EXERCISE 33 ▸ Listening. (Charts 5-6 and 5-7)
Read the information about Ben. Then complete the questions with the words you hear.

Ben's Sleeping Problem

Ben has a problem with insomnia. He's unable to fall asleep at night very easily. He also wakes up often in the middle of the night and has trouble getting back to sleep. Right now he's talking to a nurse at a sleep disorders clinic. The nurse is asking him some general questions.

1. _____ you?

2. _____ you?

3. _____ you weigh?

4. In general, _____ you sleep at night?

5. _____ you fall asleep?

6. _____ you wake up during the night?

7. _____ you in the mornings?

8. _____ you exercise?

9. _____ you feeling right now?

10. _____ you come in for an
overnight appointment?

EXERCISE 34 ▸ Warm-up. (Chart 5-8)

Look at the map and answer the questions about flying distances to these cities.

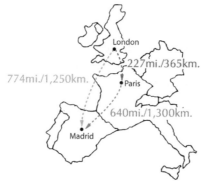

1. How far is it from London to Madrid?
2. How many miles is it from London to Paris?
3. How many kilometers is it from Paris to Madrid?

5-8 Talking About Distance

(a) *It is* 489 miles *from* Oslo *to* Helsinki by air.*	The most common way of expressing distance: **It is** + distance + **from/to** + **to/from**
(b) *It is* 3,605 miles { *from* Moscow *to* Beijing. *from* Beijing *to* Moscow. *to* Beijing *from* Moscow. *to* Moscow *from* Beijing. }	In (b): All four expressions with **from** and **to** have the same meaning.
(c) — *How far is it* from Mumbai to Delhi? — 725 miles. (d) — *How far do you* live from school? — Four blocks.	**How far** is used to ask questions about distance.
(e) *How many miles* is it from London to Paris? (f) *How many kilometers* is it to Montreal from here? (g) *How many blocks* is it to the post office?	Other ways to ask **how far**: • *how many miles* • *how many kilometers* • *how many blocks*

*1 mile = 1.60 kilometers; 1 kilometer = 0.621 mile

EXERCISE 35 ▸ Looking at grammar. (Chart 5-8)

Make questions with **How far** or **How many**.

1. A: _How far / How many miles is it from Prague to Budapest?_
   B: 276 miles. (It's 276 miles to Prague from Budapest.)

2. A: _____
   B: 257 kilometers. (It's 257 kilometers from Montreal to Quebec.)

3. A: _____
   B: Six blocks. (It's six blocks from here to the post office.)

4. A: _____

   B: A few miles. (It's a few miles from work to here.)

EXERCISE 36 ▶ Grammar and speaking. (Chart 5-8)
Ask about distances between major cities. Write four questions. Use this model: ***How far is it from (__) to (__)?*** Look up the correct distances in miles and kilometers. Ask other students your questions, and have them guess the answers.

Example: Cairo (Egypt) \ New Delhi (India) Answer: (4,438 km/2,758 miles)
STUDENT A: How far is it from Cairo to New Delhi?
STUDENT B: It's 4,000 kilometers.
STUDENT A: Almost!/Not bad!/Pretty good! It's about 4,400 kilometers.

EXERCISE 37 ▶ Warm-up. (Chart 5-9)
Complete the sentences. Then ask classmates about their weekday routine. Begin with ***How long does it take you to***. Share some of their answers with the class.

1. It takes me _____ minutes to get ready for bed.

2. It takes me _____ minutes to brush my teeth.

3. It usually takes me _____ minutes/hour(s) to fall asleep.

4. It takes me _____ minutes/hour(s) to get ready in the morning.

5. It takes me _____ minutes/hour(s) to get to school.

5-9	Length of Time: *It + Take* and *How Long; How Many*	
IT + TAKE + (SOMEONE) + LENGTH OF TIME + INFINITIVE		**It + take** is often used with time words and an infinitive to express *length of time,* as in (a) and (b).
(a) *It* takes 20 minutes *to cook* rice.		
(b) *It* took Al two hours *to drive* to work.		An infinitive = **to** + *the simple form of a verb.** In (a): **to cook** is an infinitive.
(c) *How long* does it take to cook rice? Twenty minutes. (d) *How long* did it take Al to drive to work today? Two hours. (e) *How long* did you study last night? Four hours. (f) *How long* will you be in Hong Kong? Ten days.		**How long** asks about *length of time.*
(g) *How many days* will you be in Hong Kong?		Other ways of asking **how long:** **how many** + { minutes / hours / days / weeks / months / years }

*See Chart 13-3, p. 374.

Work with a partner. Take turns asking and answering questions using *it + take*. Share a few of your answers with the class.

1. How long does it take you to …
    a. eat breakfast? → *It takes me ten minutes to eat breakfast.*
    b. take a shower?
    c. get to class?
    d. write a short paragraph in English?
    e. read a 300-page book?
    f. clean your room?

2. In general, how long does it take to …
    a. fly from (*a city*) to (*a city*)?
    b. get from here to your hometown?
    c. get used to living in a foreign country?
    d. get a visa?
    e. commute from (*a local place*) to (*a local place*) during rush hour?
    f. learn English well?

EXERCISE 39 ▸ Looking at grammar. (Chart 5-9)

Part I. Make questions with *How many*.

1. A: _____
   B: Five days. (It took me five days to drive to Istanbul.)

2. A: _____
   B: A week. (Mr. McNally will be in the hospital for a week.)

3. A: _____
   B: Six months. (I've been living here for six months.)

Part II. Make questions with *How long*.

4. A: _____
   B: Ten years. (I lived in Oman for six years.)

5. A: _____
   B: A long time. (It takes a long time to learn a second language.)

6. A: _____
   B: A couple of years. (I've known Mr. Pham for a couple of years.)

7. A: _____
   B: Since 2005. (He's been living in Canada since 2005.)

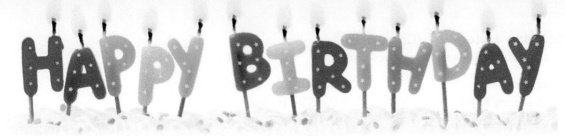

EXERCISE 40 ▶ Warm-up: listening. (Chart 5-10)

Listen to the questions. The question words and verbs in green are contracted. Choose the correct verb in the box for each question.

does	did	is	are	will

A Birthday

1. When's your birthday? _____

2. When'll your party be? _____

3. Where'd you decide to have it? _____

4. Who're you inviting? _____

5-10 Spoken and Written Contractions with Question Words

	Spoken	
is	(a) "*When's* he coming?" "*Why's* she late?"	**Is, are, does, did, has, have,** and **will** are often contracted with question words in spoken English.
are	(b) "*What're* these?" "*Who're* they talking to?"	
does	(c) "*When's* the movie start?" "*Where's* he live?"	
did	(d) "*Who'd* you see?" "*What'd* you do?"	
has	(e) "*What's* she done?" "*Where's* he gone?"	
have	(f) "*How've* you been?" "*What've* I done?"	
will	(g) "*Where'll* you be?" "*When'll* they be here?"	
	(h) *What do you* → *Whaddaya* think? (i) *What are you* → *Whaddaya* thinking?	**What do you** and **What are you** both can be reduced to *Whaddaya* in informal speech.
	Written	
is	(j) *Where's* Ed? *What's* that? *Who's* he?	Only contractions with **where, what,** or **who** + **is** are commonly used in writing — in text messages and emails, for example. They are generally not appropriate in more formal writing, such as in magazine articles or reference material.

EXERCISE 41 ▸ Listening. (Chart 5-10)
Listen to the contractions in these questions.

1. Where is my key?
2. Where are my keys?
3. Who are those people?
4. What is in that box?
5. What are you doing?
6. Where did Bob go last night?
7. Who will be at the party?

8. Why is the teacher absent?
9. Who is that?
10. Why did you say that?
11. Who did you talk to at the party?
12. How are we going to get to work?
13. What did you say?
14. How will you do that?

EXERCISE 42 ▸ Grammar and listening. (Chart 5-10)
Write the full form of the verb in the contractions: *is*, *are*, *does*, *did*, and *will*. Then listen to the sentences and note the pronunciation of the contractions.

On an Airplane

Examples: You will hear: When's the plane taking off?
You will write: _____*is*_____

You will hear: When's the plane land?
You will write: _____*does*_____

1. Who're you going to sit with? _____

2. How're you going to get your bag under the seat? _____

3. What'd the flight attendant just say? _____

4. Why'd we need to put our seat belts back on? _____

5. Why's the plane descending? _____

6. Why's the flight attendant look worried? _____

7. When'll the pilot tell us what's going on? _____

8. Why're we landing now? _____

9. Who'll meet you when you land? _____

10. When's our connecting flight? _____

11. How'll we get from the airport to our hotel? _____

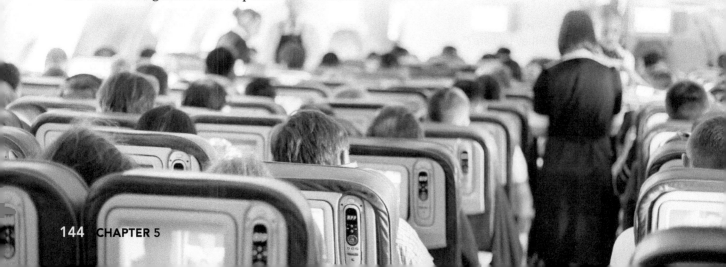

EXERCISE 43 ▶ Listening. (Chart 5-10)
Complete the questions with the words you hear. Write the non-contracted or non-reduced forms.

A Mother Talking to Her Teenage Daughter

1. _____ going?
2. _____ going with?
3. _____ that?
4. _____ known him?
5. _____ meet him?
6. _____ go to school?
7. _____ a good student?
8. _____ be back?
9. _____ wearing that outfit?
10. _____ giving me that look?
11. _____ asking so many questions?

Because I love you!

EXERCISE 44 ▶ Listening. (Chart 5-10)
Listen to the questions and circle the correct non-reduced forms of the words you hear.

Example: You will hear: Whaddaya want?

You will choose: What are you   (What do you)

1. What are you	What do you	5. What are you	What do you
2. What are you	What do you	6. What are you	What do you
3. What are you	What do you	7. What are you	What do you
4. What are you	What do you	8. What are you	What do you

EXERCISE 45 ▶ Warm-up. (Chart 5-11)
Part I. Both sentences in each pair are grammatically correct. Which question in each pair do you think is more common in spoken English?

1. a. How do you spell *Hawaii*?
   b. What is the spelling for *Hawaii*?

2. a. How do you pronounce G-A-R-A-G-E?
   b. What is the pronunciation for G-A-R-A-G-E?

Part II. Which two questions have the same meaning?

1. How are you doing?
2. How's it going?
3. How do you do?

5-11 More Questions with *How*

Question		Answer
(a) *How do you spell* "coming"?	C-O-M-I-N-G.	To answer (a): Spell the word.
(b) *How do you say* "yes" in Japanese?	Hai.	To answer (b): Say the word.
(c) *How do you say / pronounce* this word?	_____	To answer (c): Pronounce the word.
(d) *How are you getting along?* (e) *How are you doing?* (f) *How's it going?*	Great. Fine. OK. So-so.	In (d), (e), and (f): How is your life? Is your life OK? Do you have any problems? NOTE: Example (f) is also used in greetings: *Hi, Bob. How's it going?*
(g) *How do you feel?* *How are you feeling?*	Terrific! Wonderful! Great! Fine. OK. So-so. A bit under the weather. Not so good. Terrible! / Lousy. / Awful!	The questions in (g) ask about health or about general emotional state.
(h) *How do you do?*	How do you do?	In (h): ***How do you do?*** is used by two speakers when they meet each other for the first time in a very formal situation.*

*A: *Dr. Erickson, I'd like to introduce you to a friend of mine, Rick Brown. Rick, this is my biology professor, Dr. Erickson.*
 B: ***How do you do,** Mr. Brown?*
 C: ***How do you do,** Dr. Erickson? I'm pleased to meet you.*

EXERCISE 46 ▶ Game. (Chart 5-11)

Divide into teams. Take turns spelling the words your teacher gives you. The team with the most correct answers wins. Your book is closed.

Example: country
TEACHER: How do you spell *country*?
TEAM A: C-O-U-N-T-R-Y.
TEACHER: Good.
            (*If the answer is incorrect, another team tries.*)

1. together	9. beginning
2. people	10. intelligent
3. daughter	11. Mississippi
4. beautiful	12. purple
5. foreign	13. rained
6. neighbor	14. different
7. happened	15. wonderful
8. awful	16. computer

EXERCISE 47 ▸ Let's talk. (Chart 5-11)

Walk around the room and ask your classmates how to say each word or phrase in another language (Japanese, Arabic, German, French, Korean, etc.). If someone doesn't know, ask another person. Use this question: ***How do you say*** (__) in (__)?

Example:

STUDENT: A: How do you say *yes* in French?
STUDENT: B: *Yes* in French is *oui*.

1. No.
2. Thank you.
3. OK.
4. How are you?
5. Good-bye.
6. Excuse me.

EXERCISE 48 ▸ Let's talk: interview. (Chart 5-11)

Walk around the room. Interview your classmates. Practice the following questions: ***How are you doing? / How's it going? / How do you feel? / How are you feeling?*** Use the answers in Chart 5-11, section (g).

EXERCISE 49 ▸ Warm-up. (Chart 5-12)

In the conversation, the speakers are making suggestions. <u>Underline</u> their suggestions.

A: Let's invite the Thompsons over for dinner.

B: Good idea! How about next Sunday?

A: Let's do it sooner. What about this Saturday?

5-12 Using *How About* and *What About*

(a) A: We need one more player. B: *How about / What about Jack?* Let's ask him if he wants to play.	***How about*** and ***what about*** have the same meaning and usage. They are used to make suggestions or offers.
(b) A: What time should we meet? B: *How about / What about three o'clock?*	***How about*** and ***what about*** are followed by a noun (or pronoun) or the ***-ing*** form of a verb (gerund).
(c) A: What should we do this afternoon? B: *How about going* to the zoo?	NOTE: ***How about*** and ***what about*** are frequently used in informal spoken English, but are usually not used in writing.
(d) A: *What about asking* Sally over for dinner next Sunday? B: OK. Good idea.	
(e) A: I'm tired. *How about you?* B: Yes, I'm tired too.	***How about you?*** and ***What about you?*** are used to ask a question that refers to the information or question that immediately preceded it.
(f) A: Are you hungry? B: No. *What about you?* A: I'm a little hungry.	In (e): ***How about you?*** = ***Are you tired?*** In (f): ***What about you?*** = ***Are you hungry?***

EXERCISE 50 ▶ Grammar and listening. (Chart 5-12)
Choose the best response. Then listen to each conversation and check your answer.

Example:
SPEAKER A: What are you going to do over vacation?
SPEAKER B: I'm staying here. What about you?
SPEAKER A: a. Yes, I will. I have a vacation too.
            (b.) I'm going to Jordan to visit my sister.
            c. I did too.

1. A: Did you like the movie?
   B: It was OK, I guess. How about you?
   A: a. I thought it was pretty good.
        b. I'm sure.
        c. I saw it last night.

2. A: Are you going to the company party?
   B: I haven't decided yet. What about you?
   A: a. I didn't know that.
        b. Why am I going?
        c. I think I will.

3. A: Do you like living in this city?
   B: Sort of. How about you?
   A: a. I'm living in the city.
        b. I'm not sure. It's pretty noisy.
        c. Yes, I have been.

4. A: What are you going to have?
   B: Well, I'm not really hungry. I think I might just order a salad. How about you?
   A: a. I'll have one too.
        b. I'm eating at a restaurant.
        c. No, I'm not.

EXERCISE 51 ▶ Let's talk: pairwork. (Chart 5-12)
Here are some questions you can use to begin conversations. Use them to make short conversations with a partner. You can look at your book before you speak. When you speak, look at your partner.

Example:
PARTNER A: What kind of movies do you like to watch?
PARTNER B: I like comedies. I like to laugh. How about/What about you?
PARTNER A: Thrillers are my favorite. I just saw (*name of movie*). It was so exciting. Have you seen it?
PARTNER B: Yes, I really enjoyed it. My favorite part was…

1. How long have you been living in (*this city or country*)?
2. What are you going to do after class today?
3. Vacation is coming up soon. What are your plans?

Change roles.

4. How is school/are your classes going for you?
5. How often do you speak English outside of class?
6. How has your day been so far?

What is the <u>expected</u> response? Circle *yes* or *no*.

1. You're studying English, aren't you?   Yes.   No.

2. You're not a native speaker of English, are you?   Yes.   No.

5-13 Tag Questions

(a) Jill is sick, *isn't she?* (b) You didn't know, *did you?* (c) There's enough time, *isn't there?* (d) I'm not late, *am I?* (e) I'm late, *aren't I?*	A tag question is a question that is added on to the end of a sentence. An auxiliary verb is used in a tag question. Note that **I am** becomes **aren't I** in a negative tag, as in (e). (*Am I not* is also possible, but it is very formal and rare.)

Affirmative (+)	Negative (−)	Affirmative (+) Expected Answer	When the main verb is affirmative, the tag question is negative, and the expected answer agrees with the main verb.
(f) *You know* Bill,	*don't you?*	Yes.	
(g) *Marie is* from Paris,	*isn't she?*	Yes.	

Negative (−)	Affirmative (+)	Negative (−) Expected Answer	When the main verb is negative, the tag question is affirmative, and the expected answer agrees with the main verb.
(h) *You don't know* Tom,	*do you?*	No.	
(i) *Marie isn't* from Athens,	*is she?*	No.	

THE SPEAKER'S QUESTION	THE SPEAKER'S IDEA
	Tag questions have two types of intonation: rising and falling. The intonation determines the meaning of the tag.
(j) It will be nice tomorrow, *won't it?*	A speaker uses rising intonation to make sure information is correct. In (j): The speaker has an idea; the speaker is checking to see if the idea is correct.
(k) It will be nice tomorrow, *won't it?*	Falling intonation is used when the speaker is seeking agreement. In (k): The speaker thinks it will be nice tomorrow and is almost certain the listener will agree.
YES/NO QUESTIONS (l) — Will it be nice tomorrow? — Yes, it will. OR No, it won't.	In (l): The speaker has no idea. The speaker is simply looking for information. Compare (j) and (k) with (l).

 EXERCISE 53 ▶ Listening and grammar. (Chart 5-13)
Listen to each pair of sentences and answer the question.

1. a. You're Mrs. Rose, aren't you?
   b. Are you Mrs. Rose?

   QUESTION: In which sentence is the speaker checking to see if her information is correct?

2. a. Do you take cream with your coffee?

   b. You take cream with your coffee, don't you?

   QUESTION: In which sentence does the speaker have no idea?

3. a. You don't want to leave, do you?

   b. Do you want to leave?

   QUESTION: In which sentence is the speaker looking for agreement?

EXERCISE 54 ▸ Grammar and listening. (Chart 5-13)
Complete the tag questions with the correct verbs. Then listen to the questions and check your answers.

1. **SIMPLE PRESENT**

   a. You *like* strong coffee, _____*don't*_____ you?

   b. David *goes* to Ames High School, _____ he?

   c. Leila and Sara *live* on Tree Road, _____ they?

   d. Jane *has* the keys to the storeroom, _____ she?

   e. Jane's in her office, _____ she?

   f. You're a member of this class, _____ you?

   g. Oleg *doesn't have* a car, _____ he?

   h. Lisa *isn't* from around here, _____ she?

   i. I'm in trouble, _____ I?

2. **SIMPLE PAST**

   a. Paul *went* to Indonesia, _____ he?

   b. You *didn't talk* to the boss, _____ you?

   c. Ted's parents *weren't* at home, _____ they?

   d. That *was* Pat's idea, _____ it?

3. **PRESENT PROGRESSIVE, *BE GOING TO*, AND PAST PROGRESSIVE**

   a. You're *studying* hard, _____ you?

   b. Greg *isn't working* at the bank, _____ he?

   c. It *isn't going to rain* today, _____ it?

   d. Michelle and Yoko *were helping*, _____ they?

   e. He *wasn't listening*, _____ he?

4. **PRESENT PERFECT**

   a. It *has been* warmer than usual, _____ it?

   b. You've *had* a lot of homework, _____ you?

   c. We *haven't spent* much time together, _____ we?

d. Fatima *has started* her new job, _____ she?

e. Bruno *hasn't finished* his sales report yet, _____ he?

f. Steve's *had to leave* early, _____ he?

EXERCISE 55 ▸ Let's talk: pairwork. (Chart 5-13)

Work with a partner. Make true statements for your partner to agree with. Remember, if your partner makes an affirmative statement before the tag, the expected answer is *yes*. If your partner makes a negative statement before the tag, the expected answer is *no*.

1. The weather is _____ today, isn't it?

2. This book costs _____, doesn't it?

3. I'm _____, aren't I?

4. The classroom isn't _____, is it?

5. Our grammar homework wasn't _____, was it?

6. Tomorrow will be _____, won't it?

EXERCISE 56 ▸ Listening. (Chart 5-13)

Listen to the tag questions and choose the <u>expected responses</u>.

Checking in at a Hotel

Example: You will hear: Our room's ready, isn't it?
You will choose: (Yes.)   No.

1. Yes.   No.   6. Yes.   No.

2. Yes.   No.   7. Yes.   No.

3. Yes.   No.   8. Yes.   No.

4. Yes.   No.   9. Yes.   No.

5. Yes.   No.   10. Yes.   No.

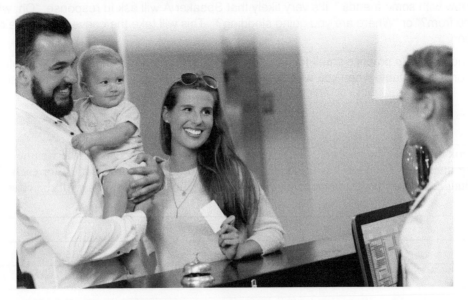

EXERCISE 57 ▸ Reading and speaking. (Chapter 5 Review)

Part I. Read the blog entry by co-author Stacy Hagen.

BlackBookBlog

Do you know these words?
- casual
- challenging
- acceptable
- politics
- likely

Small Talk

Small talk (light casual conversation for informal situations) can be challenging in any language, but it is particularly difficult for nonnative speakers. Every culture has topics that are acceptable for small talk. In English-speaking countries, it is common to talk about the weather. This is a very safe topic. An unsafe topic would be politics. People can have strong feelings about political topics and may get into arguments.

Here are some common conversation starters about the weather:
   Beautiful day, isn't it?
   Have you ever seen so much rain/snow/ice?
   Are you enjoying this beautiful day/sunny day/sunshine?
   I'm really enjoying the sun this week. How about you?

A helpful hint is to always add a detail when you answer. This will help keep the conversation going. For example:

   A: Beautiful day, isn't?
   B: Yes, I'm really enjoying the sunshine. <u>I'm not from here, and this much sun is a nice surprise.</u>

   OR

   A: Have you ever seen so much snow?
   B: No, I haven't. But it's really fun. <u>I'm going to go sledding tomorrow with some friends.</u>

Note that Speaker B added the detail "I'm not from here, … " or "I'm going to go sledding tomorrow with some friends." It's very likely that Speaker A will ask in response, "Oh, where are you from?" or "Where are you going sledding?" This will take the conversation in a new direction.

It is a good idea to practice small-talk starters so you can get better at them. It will help you feel more comfortable when you want to start a conversation with someone for the first time.

Part II. Look outside at the weather. Write three conversation starters about the weather. Use at least one tag question. Then work with a partner and create a short conversation for each. Remember to add a detail in Partner B's first response. Share one of your conversations with the class.

A: _____

B: _____

A: _____

B: _____

EXERCISE 58 ▸ Listening and speaking. (Chapter 5 Review)
Part I. Listen to the conversation. A customer is ordering at a fast-food restaurant.

Ordering at a Fast-Food Restaurant

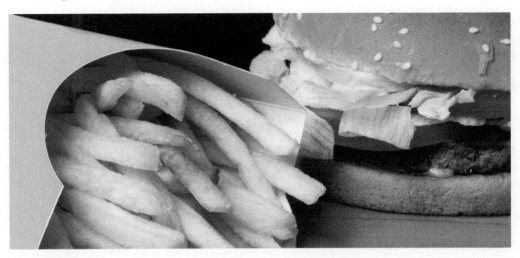

Part II. Work with a partner. Take turns being the cashier and the customer. Complete the sentences with items from the menu and practice your conversation.

burger	chicken strips	soft drinks: *cola, lemon soda, iced tea*
cheeseburger	fish burger	milkshakes: *vanilla, strawberry, chocolate*
double cheeseburger	veggie burger	*(small, medium, large)*
fries	salad	

CASHIER: So, what'll it be?

CUSTOMER: I'll have a _____.

CASHIER: Would you like fries or a salad with your burger?

CUSTOMER: I'll have (a) _____.

CASHIER: What size?

CUSTOMER: _____.

CASHIER: Anything to drink?

CUSTOMER: I'll have a _____.

CASHIER: Size?

CUSTOMER: _____.

CASHIER: OK. So that's _____
_____.

CUSTOMER: About how long'll it take?

CASHIER: We're pretty crowded right now. Probably 10 minutes or so. That'll be $6.50.

Your number's on the receipt. I'll call the number when your order's ready.

CUSTOMER: Thanks.

EXERCISE 59 ▸ Check your knowledge. (Chapter 5 Review)

Correct the errors in question formation.

1. Who you saw? → *Who did you see?*

2. Where I buy subway tickets?

3. What for you are leaving?

4. What kind of tea you like best?

5. It's freezing out, and you're not wearing gloves, aren't you?

6. Who you studied with at school?

7. She is going to work this weekend, doesn't she?

8. How long take to get to the airport from here?

9. How much height your father have?

10. It's midnight. Why you so late? Why you forget to call?

EXERCISE 60 ▸ Writing (Chapter 5)

Part I. Read the text messages. Note the variety of questions in J's response.

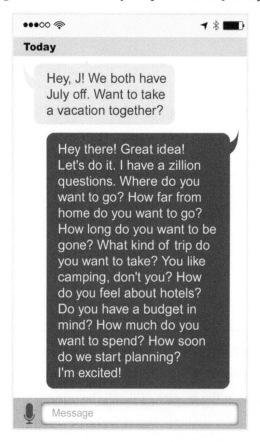

Part II. Imagine that you are going to visit a friend in another country. You decide the country — one you have never visited. What kinds of things do you need to know before you go? Respond to your friend's text message and ask a variety of questions.

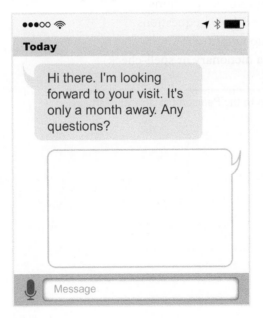

WRITING TIP

It is easy to confuse *what* and *how* when you write or ask questions. Since you are probably more familiar with *what* questions, here are some general guidelines for *how* questions:

1. *How* is used with adjectives or adverbs:

   How + far / tall / old / fast / cold / often / long / soon / late / big / much / many

   How far do you want to go?
   How soon do you want to leave?

2. *How* is used in greetings and to ask for opinions:

   How are you doing?
   How have you been?
   How do you feel about … ?
   How do you like … ?

3. *How* is used for weather and transportation:

   How is the weather?
   How will we get there?

Watch out for these commonly confused questions with *how* and *what*:

CORRECT: How do you know?	INCORRECT: Why do you know?
CORRECT: What do you think?	INCORRECT: How do you think?
CORRECT: What do you call this?	INCORRECT: How do you call this?

Part III. Edit your writing. Check for the following:

1. ☐ correct question word order
2. ☐ correct use of helping verbs in questions
3. ☐ correct use of *what* and *how* in questions
4. ☐ use of different question types
5. ☐ correct spelling (use a dictionary or spell-check)

■■■■■ For digital resources, go to the Pearson Practice English app.

CHAPTER 6
Nouns and Pronouns

PRETEST: What do I already know?
Write "C" if the **boldfaced** words are correct and "I" if they are incorrect.

1. _____ There are many interesting **citys** in Asia. (Chart 6-1)

2. _____ My mom and grandma are very strong **women**. (Chart 6-1)

3. _____ **Shines the sun**. (Chart 6-3)

4. _____ I left your **phone the kitchen counter**. (Chart 6-4)

5. _____ I study English **in the night**. (Chart 6-5)

6. _____ I left **in 2015 my country**. (Chart 6-6)

7. _____ Every person in the world **needs** love. (Chart 6-7)

8. _____ Montreal and Vancouver are **places beautifuls** to visit. (Chart 6-8)

9. _____ I want to show you my **vegetables garden**. (Chart 6-9)

10. _____ This summer, my friend Mira is going to visit **my sister and me**. (Chart 6-10)

11. _____ The **two brother houses** look identical. (Chart 6-11)

12. _____ **Whose** backpack is this? (Chart 6-12)

13. _____ You have your beliefs, and I have **my**. (Chart 6-13)

14. _____ Greta's husband forgets her birthday, so she buys **herself** a present every year. (Chart 6-14)

15. _____ I brought two oranges. Do you want this one, and I'll have **other** one? (Chart 6-15)

16. _____ Green and red are not my favorite colors. Do you have this shirt in **other** colors?

EXERCISE 1 ▶ Warm-up. (Chart 6-1)
Write *one* if the noun is singular. Write *two* if the noun is plural.

In the Kitchen

1. _____ onion

2. _____ spices

3. _____ tomato

4. _____ berries

5. _____ dishes

6. _____ knives

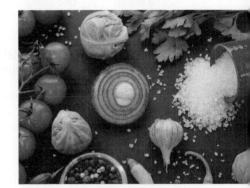

6-1 Plural Forms of Nouns

Singular	Plural	
(a) one bird one street one rose	two *birds* two *streets* two *roses*	SINGULAR = one PLURAL = more than one To make most nouns plural, add **-s**.
(b) one dish one match one class one box	two *dishes* two *matches* two *classes* two *boxes*	Add **-es** to nouns ending in **-sh**, **-ch**, **-ss**, and **-x**.
(c) one baby one city	two *babies* two *cities*	If a noun ends in a consonant + **-y**, change the **y** to **i** and add **-es**, as in (c).
(d) one toy one key	two *toys* two *keys*	If **-y** is preceded by a vowel, add only **-s**, as in (d).
(e) one knife one shelf	two *knives* two *shelves*	If a noun ends in **-fe** or **-f,** change the ending to **-ves**. EXCEPTIONS: *beliefs, chiefs, roofs, cuffs, cliffs.*

(f) one tomato
one zoo
one zero
	two *tomatoes*
	two *zoos*
	two *zeroes/zeros*
		The plural form of nouns that end in **-o** is sometimes **-oes** and sometimes **-os**.
		-oes: *tomatoes, potatoes, heroes*
		-os: *zoos, radios, studios, pianos, solos, sopranos, photos,*
		      autos, videos
		-oes or **-os**: *zeroes/zeros, volcanoes/volcanos, tornadoes/tornados,*
		      mosquitoes/mosquitos, echoes/echos

(g) one child one foot one goose one man one mouse one tooth one woman _____	two *children* two *feet* two *geese* two *men* two *mice* two *teeth* two *women* two *people*	Some nouns have irregular plural forms. NOTE: The singular form of *people* can be *person, woman, man, child*. For example, one *man* and one *child* = two *people*. (Two *persons* is also possible, but not very common.)
(h) one deer one fish one sheep	two *deer* two *fish* two *sheep*	Some nouns may have the same singular and plural forms.

EXERCISE 2 ▸ Looking at grammar. (Chart 6-1)

Write the correct singular or plural form for each noun.

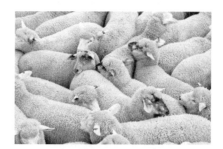

1. one chair   two _____*chairs*_____

2. a _____   a lot of windows

3. one wish   several _____

4. one _____   a lot of sheep

5. a tax   a lot of _____

6. one boy   two _____

7. a hobby   several _____

8. one leaf   two _____

9. a _____ two halves

10. a belief   many _____

11. one wolf   two _____

12. a radio   several _____

13. one _____ two feet

14. an _____ two addresses

EXERCISE 3 ▸ Game. (Chart 6-1)

Work in teams. Write the plural form of each noun under the correct heading. The number of words for each column is in parentheses. NOTE: **fish** and **thief** can go in two places.

✓butterfly	child	hero	mouse	thief
baby	city	library	✓museum	tomato
boy	fish	✓man	potato	woman
✓bean	girl	mosquito	sandwich	zoo

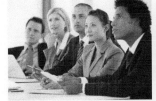 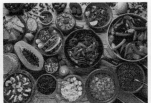 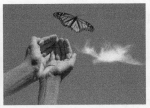 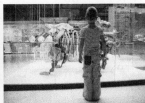

PEOPLE (8)	FOOD (5)	THINGS PEOPLE CATCH (5)	PLACES PEOPLE VISIT (4)
men	*beans*	*butterflies*	*museums*

EXERCISE 4 ▸ Looking at grammar. (Chart 6-1)

Part I. Edit the sign by giving the appropriate nouns their correct plural forms. There are eight errors.

ON SALE

(while supply last)

shirt   jean   pant   dress

Outfit and shoe for babys 50% off

Part II. Imagine you are selling some items online that you don't need any longer. Write an ad and list eight items you would like to sell. Make sure that some of your items are plural.

EXERCISE 5 ▸ Warm-up: listening. (Chart 6-2)
Listen to the nouns. Circle *yes* if you hear a plural ending. If not, circle *no*.

Examples: You will hear: books
             You will choose: (yes)   no

             You will hear: class
             You will choose: yes   (no)

1. yes	no	3. yes	no	5. yes	no
2. yes	no	4. yes	no	6. yes	no

6-2 Pronunciation of Final -s/-es

Final **-s/-es** has three different pronunciations: /s/, /z/, and / əz/.

(a)	seats = seat/s/ maps = map/s/ lakes = lake/s/	Final **-s** is pronounced /s/ after voiceless sounds. In (a): /s/ is the sound of "s" in *bus*. Examples of voiceless* sounds: /t/, /p/, /k/.
(b)	seeds = seed/z/ stars = star/z/ holes = hole/z/ laws = law/z/	Final **-s** is pronounced /z/ after voiced sounds. In (b): /z/ is the sound of "z" in *buzz*. Examples of voiced* sounds: /d/, /r/, /l/, /m/, /b/, and all vowel sounds.
(c)	dishes = dish/əz/ matches = match/əz/ classes = class/əz/ sizes = size/əz/ pages = page/əz/ judges = judge/əz/	Final **-s/-es** is pronounced /əz/ after -sh, -ch, -s, -z, -ge/-dge sounds. In (c): /əz/ adds a syllable to a word.

*See Appendix A-6 for more information about voiceless and voiced sounds.

EXERCISE 6 ▸ Listening. (Chart 6-2)
Listen to the words. Circle the sound you hear at the end of each word: /s/, /z/, or /əz/.

1. pan**ts**   /s/   /z/   /əz/

2. car**s**   /s/   /z/   /əz/

3. box**es**   /s/   /z/   /əz/

4. pen**s**   /s/   /z/   /əz/

5. wish**es**   /s/   /z/   /əz/

6. lak**es**   /s/   /z/   /əz/

EXERCISE 7 ▸ Listening. (Chart 6-2)
Listen to each pair of words. Decide if the endings have the same sound or a different sound.

Examples: You will hear: maps   streets
You will choose: (same)   different

You will hear: knives   forks
You will choose: same   (different)

1. same   different   5. same   different

2. same   different   6. same   different

3. same   different   7. same   different

4. same   different   8. same   different

EXERCISE 8 ▸ Listening and pronunciation. (Chart 6-2)
Listen to the words. Write the pronunciation of each ending you hear: /s/, /z/, or /əz/. After you correct the answers, practice pronouncing the words.

1. names = name/z/   4. boats = boat/ /   7. lips = lip/ /

2. clocks = clock/s/   5. eyelashes = eyelash/ /   8. bridges = bridge/ /

3. eyes = eye/ /   6. ways = way/ /   9. cars = car/ /

EXERCISE 9 ▸ Listening. (Chart 6-2)
Listen to the sentences and circle the words you hear. Practice pronouncing them.

1. size   sizes   3. tax   taxes   5. glass   glasses

2. tax   taxes   4. price   prices   6. prize   prizes

EXERCISE 10 ▸ Warm-up. (Chart 6-3)
Part I. Work in small groups. Make lists about the topic of friendship.

1. What qualities are important in a friendship?
2. Name things you do with friends.
3. What social media do you use to stay connected to friends?

Part II. Complete the sentences with information from Part I. Share some of your sentences with the class.

1. _____ and _____ are important qualities in a friendship.

2. I _____ and _____ with my friends.

3. I use _____ to stay connected to friends.

Part III. Answer these questions about your answers in Part II.

1. In which sentence did you write verbs?
2. In which two sentences did you write nouns?
3. In which sentence did you write subjects?
4. In which sentence did you write objects?

6-3 Subjects, Verbs, and Objects

(a) The	S *sun* (noun)	V *shines.* (verb)	An English sentence has a SUBJECT (S) and a VERB (V). The SUBJECT is a *noun*. In (a): **sun** is a noun; it is the subject of the verb **shines**.
(b)	S *Plants* (noun)	V *grow.* (verb)	NOTE: Some nouns can also be verbs: People **plant** flowers.
(c)	S *Plants* (noun)	V *need* (verb)	O *water.* (noun)	Sometimes a VERB is followed by an OBJECT (O). The OBJECT of a verb is a *noun*. In (c): **water** is the object of the verb **need**. An object answers the question *What?* *What do plants need?* *What is Bob reading?*
(d)	S *Bob* (noun)	V *is reading* (verb)	O *a book.* (noun)	

EXERCISE 11 ▶ Looking at grammar. (Chart 6-3)

Complete each diagram with the correct subject, verb, and object.

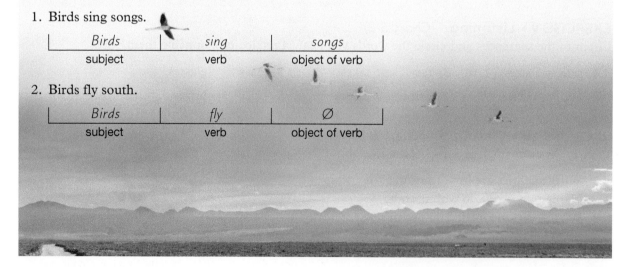

1. Birds sing songs.

Birds	*sing*	*songs*
subject	verb	object of verb

2. Birds fly south.

Birds	*fly*	Ø
subject	verb	object of verb

3. Birds build nests.

subject	verb	object of verb

4. The sun heats the earth.

subject	verb	object of verb

5. The sun sets at night.

subject	verb	object of verb

6. The moon rises every evening.

subject	verb	object of verb

7. Fires destroy forests.

subject	verb	object of verb

8. Surprises happen every day.

subject	verb	object of verb

EXERCISE 12 ▶ Looking at grammar. (Chart 6-3)
Write "N" if the word in green is a noun. Write "V" if it is a verb.

1. a. People smile when they're happy. _____

   b. Maryam has a nice smile when she's happy. _____

2. a. Please don't sign your name in pencil. _____

   b. People often name their children after relatives. _____

3. a. Airplanes land on runways at the airport. _____

   b. The land across the street from our house is vacant. _____

4. a. People usually store milk in the refrigerator. _____

   b. We went to the store to buy some milk. _____

5. a. I took the express train from New York to Boston
      last week. _____

   b. Lindsey trains horses as a hobby. _____

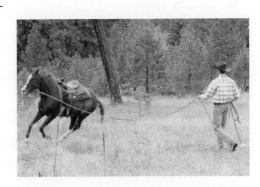

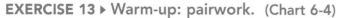

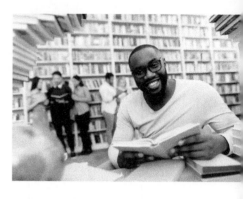

EXERCISE 13 ▶ Warm-up: pairwork. (Chart 6-4)
Work with a partner. Make true sentences about yourself using *like* or *don't like*. Share a few of your partner's answers with the class.

I like/don't like to do my homework …

1. at the library.
2. at the kitchen table.
3. in my bedroom.
4. on my bed.
5. with a friend.
6. in the evening.
7. on weekends.
8. after dinner.
9. before class.
10. during class.

6-4 Objects of Prepositions

	S	V	O	PREP	O OF PREP
(a)	Ann put her books			*on*	*the* *desk*. (noun)

Many English sentences have prepositional phrases. In (a): **on the desk** is a prepositional phrase.

	S	V	PREP	O OF PREP
(b)	A leaf fell		*to*	*the* *ground*. (noun)

A prepositional phrase consists of a PREPOSITION (PREP) and an OBJECT OF A PREPOSITION (O of PREP). The object of a preposition is a NOUN.

Reference List of Prepositions

about	before	despite	next to	to
above	behind	down	of	toward(s)
across	below	during	off	under
after	beneath	for	on	until/till*
against	beside	from	out	up
along	besides	in	over	upon
among	between	into	since	with
around	beyond	like	through	within
at	by	near	throughout	without

*Till is a more informal way of saying *until*.

EXERCISE 14 ▶ Looking at grammar. (Chart 6-4)
Check (✓) the prepositional phrases, and underline the noun in each phrase that is the object of the preposition.

1. __✓__ across the <u>street</u>

2. _____ in a minute

3. _____ daily

4. _____ down the hill

5. _____ next to the phone

6. _____ doing work

7. _____ in a few hours

8. _____ from my parents

EXERCISE 15 ▶ Looking at grammar. (Charts 6-3 and 6-4)
Check (✓) the sentences that have objects of prepositions. Identify the preposition (P) and the object of the preposition (Obj. of P).

At the Beach

1. a. _____ The wind blew loudly.
                        P   Obj. of P
   b. _✓_ The wind blew loudly at the beach.
                        P   Obj. of P
   c. _✓_ The wind pushed the waves onto the beach.

2. a. _____ Emma sat on the beach.

   b. _____ She watched the waves.

   c. _____ She didn't swim in the waves.

3. a. _____ An athletic woman jumped into the water.

   b. _____ She swam in the water.

   c. _____ She swam for an hour.

4. a. _____ Annika dropped her ring.

   b. _____ Annika dropped her ring in the sand.

   c. _____ Annika dropped her ring in the sand at the beach.

EXERCISE 16 ▶ Let's talk. (Chart 6-4)
Review prepositions of place by using each phrase in a complete sentence. Demonstrate the meaning of the preposition with an action while you say the sentence. Work in pairs, in small groups, or as a class.

Example: across the room → *I'm walking across the room.* OR *I'm looking across the room.*

1. above the door
2. against the wall
3. toward(s) the door
4. between two pages of my book
5. in the classroom
6. into the classroom
7. on my desk
8. at my desk
9. below the window
10. beside my book
11. near the door
12. far from the door
13. off my desk
14. out the window
15. behind me
16. through the door

EXERCISE 17 ▶ Game: trivia. (Chart 6-4)
Work in small groups. Answer the questions without looking at a map. After you finish, look at a map to check your answers.* The team with the most correct answers wins.

1. Name a country directly under Russia.
2. Name the country directly above Germany.
3. What river flows through London?

---

*See *Trivia Answers,* p. 247.

4. What is a country near Haiti?
5. Name a country next to Vietnam.
6. Name a city far from Sydney, Australia.
7. What is the country between Austria and Switzerland?
8. Name the city within Rome, Italy.
9. Name two countries that have a river between them.
10. Name a country that is across from Saudi Arabia.

EXERCISE 18 ▸ Reading and grammar. (Chart 6-4)
Read the passage and answer the questions.

Do you know these words?
- giant   - snakes
- insects   - frogs
- vines   - gorillas
- ground

THE HABITATS OF A RAIN FOREST

Rain forests have different areas where animals live. These areas are called *habitats*. Scientists have given names to the four main habitats or layers of a rain forest.

Some animals live in the tops of giant trees. The tops of these trees are much higher than the other trees, so this layer is called the *emergent* layer.* Many birds and insects live there.

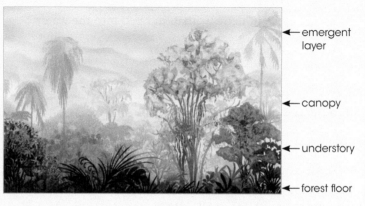

← emergent layer

← canopy

← understory

← forest floor

Under the emergent layer is the *canopy*. The canopy is the upper part of the trees. It is thick with leaves and vines, and it forms an umbrella over the rain forest. Most of the animals in the rain forest live in the canopy.

The next layer is the *understory*. The understory is above the ground and under the leaves. In the understory, it is very dark and cool. It gets only 2–5% of the sunlight that the canopy gets. The understory has the most insects of the four layers, and a lot of snakes and frogs also live there.

Finally, there is the *forest floor.* On the surface of this floor are fallen leaves, branches, and other debris.** In general, the largest animals in the rain forest live in this layer. Common animals in this habitat are tigers and gorillas.

*emergent = in botany, a plant that is taller than other plants around it, like a tall tree in a forest
**debris = loose, natural material, like dirt

1. Name two types of animals that live in the tops of giant trees.
2. What layer forms an umbrella over the rain forest?
3. Where is the understory?
4. Where do you think most mosquitoes live?
5. What are some differences between the emergent layer and the forest floor?

EXERCISE 19 ▸ Warm-up. (Chart 6-5)

Complete the sentences with information about yourself: *I was born ...*

1. in _____ (*month*).   3. on _____ (*weekday*).

2. on _____ (*date*).   4. at _____ (*time*).

6-5 Prepositions of Time

in	(a) Please be on time *in the future*. (b) I usually watch TV *in the evening*.	*in* + the past, the present, the future* *in* + the morning, the afternoon, the evening
	(c) I was born *in October*. (d) I was born *in 1995*. (e) I was born *in the 20th century*. (f) The weather is hot *in* (the) *summer*.	*in* + { a month / a year / a century / a season }
on	(g) I was born *on October 31st, 1995*. (h) I went to a movie *on Thursday*. (i) I have class *on Thursday morning(s)*.	*on* + a date *on* + a weekday *on* + (a) weekday morning(s), afternoon(s), evening(s)
at	(j) We sleep at night. I was asleep *at midnight*. (k) I fell asleep *at 9:30* (nine-thirty). (l) He's busy *at the moment*. Can I take a message?	*at* + noon, night, midnight *at* + "clock time" *at* + the moment, the present time, present

*Possible in British English: *in future* (e.g., *Please be on time in future.*)

EXERCISE 20 ▸ Looking at grammar. (Chart 6-5)

Complete the sentences with *in*, *at*, or *on*. All the sentences contain time expressions.

Studious Stan has college classes ...

1. _____ the morning.
2. _____ the afternoon.
3. _____ the evening.
4. _____ night.
5. _____ weekdays.

6. _____ Saturdays.
7. _____ Saturday mornings.
8. _____ noon.
9. _____ midnight.

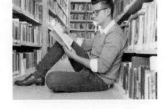

Unlucky Lisa has a birthday every four years. She was born ...

10. _____ February 29th.
11. _____ February 29th, 1976.
12. _____ February.

13. _____ 1976.
14. _____ February 1976.
15. _____ the winter.

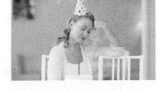

Cool Carlos is a fashion designer. He's thinking about clothing designs ...

16. _____ the moment.
17. _____ the present time.
18. _____ the past.

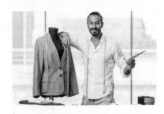

EXERCISE 21 ▸ Let's talk: interview. (Chart 6-5)

Complete each question with an appropriate preposition. Interview seven classmates. Ask each person one question. Share a few of the answers with the class.

1. What do you like to do _____ the evening?

2. What do you usually do _____ night before bed?

3. What do you like to do _____ Saturday mornings?

4. What did you do _____ January 1st of this year?

5. What were you doing _____ this time last year?

6. How do you spend your free time _____ the summer?

7. What will you do with your English skills _____ the future?

EXERCISE 22 ▸ Warm-up. (Chart 6-6)

Check (✓) all the grammatically correct sentences.

1. a. _____ I left Athens in 2005.

   b. _____ I left in 2005 Athens.

   c. _____ In 2005, I left Athens.

2. a. _____ Lee sold his car yesterday.

   b. _____ Yesterday Lee sold his car.

   c. _____ Lee sold yesterday his car.

6-6 Word Order: Place and Time

(a)   S   V   PLACE   TIME
     Mia moved *to Paris* *in 2008.*
     We went   *to a movie* *yesterday.*
	In a typical English sentence, "place" usually comes before "time," as in (a).
	 INCORRECT: *Mia moved in 2008 to Paris.*

(b)   S   V   O   P   T
     We bought a house in Miami in 2005.
	S-V-O-P-T = Subject-Verb-Object-Place-Time
	                   (basic English sentence structure)

(c) TIME S V PLACE *In 2008,* Mia moved to Paris. (d) *Yesterday* we went to a movie.	Expressions of time can also come at the beginning of a sentence, as in (c) and (d). A time phrase at the beginning of a sentence is often followed by a comma, as in (c).

EXERCISE 23 ▸ Looking at grammar. (Chart 6-6)

Put the phrases in the correct sentence order.

Updates

1. to Paris \ next month

   Monique's company is going to transfer her _____.

2. last week \ through Turkey

   William began a bike trip _____.

3. at his uncle's bakery \ Alexi \ on weekends \ works

_____.

4. am taking \ tomorrow \ a flight \ I \ to Cairo

_____.

EXERCISE 24 ▶ Warm-up. (Chart 6-7)
Add a final **-s** or **Ø**.

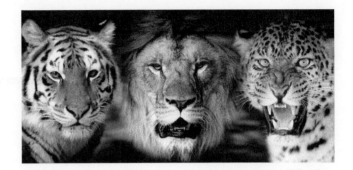

1. Lions roar_____.

2. A lion roar_____.

3. Lions, tigers, and leopards roar_____.

4. A tiger in the jungle roar_____.

5. Tigers in the jungle roar_____.

6. Tigers in jungles roar_____.

6-7 Subject-Verb Agreement

SINGULAR SINGULAR (a) The *sun* shines. PLURAL PLURAL (b) *Birds* sing.	A singular subject takes a singular verb, as in (a). A plural subject takes a plural verb, as in (b). NOTE: *verb* + **-s** = singular (*shines*) *noun* + **-s** = plural (*birds*)
SINGULAR SINGULAR (c) My *brother* lives in Jakarta. PLURAL PLURAL (d) My *brother and sister* live in Jakarta.	Two subjects connected by **and** take a plural verb, as in (d).
(e) The *glasses* over there under the window by the sink *are* clean. (f) The *information* in those magazines about Vietnamese culture and customs *is* very interesting.	Sometimes phrases come between a subject and a verb. These phrases do not affect the agreement of the subject and verb.
v s (g) *There is* a *book* on the desk. v s (h) *There are* some *books* on the desk.	**There** + **be** + *subject* expresses that something exists in a particular place. The verb agrees with the noun that follows **be**.
(i) *Every student is* sitting down. (j) *Everybody/Everyone hopes* for peace.	**Every** is a singular word. It is used with a singular, not plural, noun. *INCORRECT*: *Every students* ... Subjects with **every** take singular verbs, as in (i) and (j).
(k) *People* in my country *are* friendly.	**People** is a plural noun and takes a plural verb.

EXERCISE 25 ▶ Looking at grammar. (Chart 6-7)
Identify the subject (S) and the verb (V). Correct errors in agreement.

My Apartment Building

                                        V
            S   *are*

1. The <u>apartments</u> in this building <u>is</u> modern.

         S   V

2. Five <u>students</u> from my class <u>live</u> in this building. → OK *(no error in agreement)*

3. There is a vacant apartment in my building.

4. The people on my floor is helpful.

5. The neighbors in the apartment next to mine is very friendly.

6. My aunt and uncle live next door.

7. Every person in this building have a pet.

8. All apartments have air-conditioning.

EXERCISE 26 ▶ Looking at grammar. (Chart 6-7)
Work in small groups. Complete the sentences with the correct form of the verbs in the box.
Discuss the words you use to describe different animal sounds in your native language.

bark	buzz	scream	squeak

What sounds do these animals make?

1. A dog _____.

2. Dogs _____.

3. Monkeys and chimpanzees _____.

4. A monkey in the jungle _____.

5. Monkeys in the jungle _____.

6. A mouse and a rat _____.

7. Mice and rats _____.

8. Bees in a hive _____.

9. Every bee _____.

10. Every bee in a hive _____.

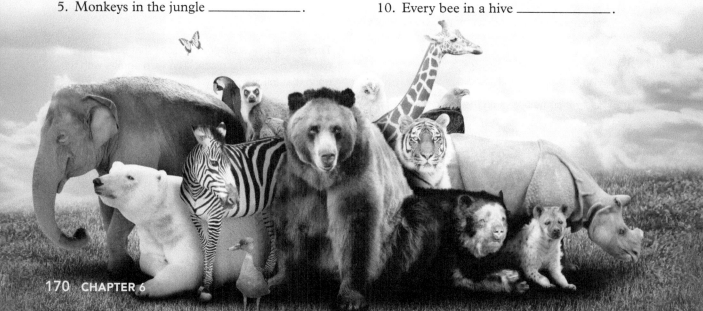

EXERCISE 27 ▶ Listening. (Charts 6-2 and 6-7)
Listen to the passage. Listen a second time and add **-s** where necessary.

Do you know these words?
- sweat   - flap
- fur   - mud
- paw

HOW SOME ANIMALS STAY COOL

How do animal_____ stay cool in hot weather? Many animal_____ don't sweat like human_____,
＿＿＿1   ＿＿＿2   ＿＿＿3

so they have other way_____ to cool themselves.
＿＿＿4

Dog_____, for example, have a lot of fur_____ and can become very hot. They stay_____ cool
＿＿＿5   ＿＿＿6   ＿＿＿7

mainly by panting. If you don't know what *panting* means, this is the sound of panting.

Cat_____ lick_____ their paw_____ and chest_____. When their fur
＿＿＿8   ＿＿＿9   ＿＿＿10   ＿＿＿11

_____ is wet, they become cooler.
＿＿＿12

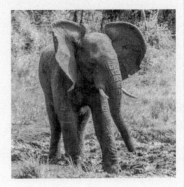

Elephant_____ have very large ear_____. When they are hot, they
＿＿＿13   ＿＿＿14

can flap their huge ear_____. The flapping ear_____ act_____ like
＿＿＿15   ＿＿＿16   ＿＿＿17

a fan, and it cool_____ them. Elephant_____ also like to roll in the
＿＿＿18   ＿＿＿19

mud_____ to stay cool.
＿＿＿20

EXERCISE 28 ▶ Warm-up. (Chart 6-8)
Think about the very first teacher you had. Choose words from below to describe him/her.

young	elderly	unfriendly	serious	impatient
middle-aged	friendly	fun	patient	helpful

6-8 Using Adjectives to Describe Nouns

ADJECTIVE NOUN (a) Rob is reading a *good* *book*.	Words that describe nouns are called ADJECTIVES. In (a): **good** is an adjective; it describes the book.
(b) The *tall* woman wore a *new* dress. (c) The *short* woman wore an *old* dress. (d) The *young* woman wore a *short* dress.	We say that adjectives "modify" nouns. *Modify* means "change a little." An adjective changes the meaning of a noun by giving more information about it.
(e) Roses are *beautiful* flowers. INCORRECT: *Roses are beautifuls flowers.*	Adjectives are neither singular nor plural. They do NOT have a plural form.
(f) He wore a *white* shirt. INCORRECT: *He wore a shirt white.* (g) Roses *are beautiful*. (h) His shirt *was white*.	Adjectives usually come immediately before nouns, as in (f). Adjectives can also follow the main verb **be**, as in (g) and (h).

EXERCISE 29 ▸ Looking at grammar. (Chart 6-8)
Check (✓) the phrases that have adjectives. Underline the adjectives.

1. __✓__ a scary story

2. _____ on Tuesday

3. _____ going to a famous place

4. _____ a small, dark, uncomfortable room

5. _____ quickly and then slowly

6 _____ long or short hair

EXERCISE 30 ▸ Looking at grammar. (Chart 6-8)
Add the given adjectives to the sentences. Only <u>two</u> of the three adjectives in each item will work.

Example: hard, heavy, strong   A man lifted the box
        → *A strong man lifted the heavy box.*

1. beautiful, safe, red   Roses are flowers.
2. empty, wet, hot   The waiter poured coffee into my cup.
3. fresh, clear, hungry   Mrs. Fields gave the kids a snack.
4. dirty, modern, delicious   After our dinner, Frank helped me with the dishes.

EXERCISE 31 ▸ Grammar and reading. (Chart 6-8)
Part I. Add your own nouns, adjectives, and prepositions to the list. Don't look at Part II.

1. an adjective _____*old*_____

2. a person's name _____

3. a plural noun _____

4. a plural noun _____

5. a singular noun _____

6. an adjective _____

7. an adjective _____

8. a preposition of place _____

9. an adjective _____

10. a plural noun _____

Part II. Complete the sentences with the same words you added in Part I. Some of your completions might sound a little odd or funny. Read your completed passage aloud to a partner, group, or the rest of the class.

    One day a/an _____*old*_____ girl was walking in the city. Her name was _____.
                    1   2
She was carrying a package for her grandmother. It had some _____, some
                                                                        3
_____, and a/an _____, among other things.
        4   5

    As she was walking down the street, a/an _____ thief stole her package.   The
                                                        6
_____ girl pulled out her cell phone and called the police, who caught the thief
        7
_____ a nearby building and returned her package to her. She took it immediately to
        8
her _____ grandmother, who was glad to get the package because she really needed
        9
some new _____.
                10

EXERCISE 32 ▸ Warm-up. (Chart 6-9)

Combine the word *chicken* with the words in the box.

✓fresh	hot	✓legs	recipe	soup

1. _____chicken legs_____
2. _____fresh chicken_____
3. _____
4. _____
5. _____

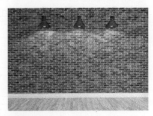

6-9 Using Nouns as Adjectives

(a) I have a *flower* garden.	Sometimes words that are usually used as nouns are used as adjectives.
(b) The *shoe* store also sells socks.	For example, *flower* is usually a noun, but in (a), it is used as an adjective to modify *garden*.
(c) INCORRECT: a flowers garden	When a noun is used as an adjective, it is singular in form, NOT plural.
(d) INCORRECT: the shoes store	

EXERCISE 33 ▸ Looking at grammar. (Chart 6-9)

Underline and identify the nouns (N). Use one of the nouns in the first sentence as an adjective in the second sentence.

1. This <u>book</u> is about <u>grammar</u>. It's a _____grammar book*_____.

2. My garden has vegetables. It's a _____.

3. The soup has beans. It's _____.

4. I read a lot of articles in magazines. I read a lot of _____.

5. The factory makes toys. It's a _____.

6. The villages are in the mountains. They are _____.

7. The lesson was about art. It was an _____.

8. Flags fly from poles. Many government buildings have _____.

9. This medicine stops coughs. I recommend this _____.

10. This wall has bricks. It's a _____.

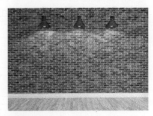

---

*When one noun modifies another noun, the spoken stress is usually on the first noun: *a **grammar** book*.

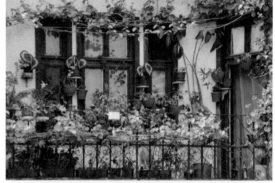

EXERCISE 34 ▶ Grammar and speaking. (Chart 6-9)

Add **-s** to the nouns in green if necessary. Then circle *yes* or *no* to agree or disagree with each sentence. Share your answers with a partner.

What do you think?

1. One day, computer programs will make it possible for computers to think.	yes	no
2. Computer make life more stressful.	yes	no
3. Airplane trips are enjoyable nowadays.	yes	no
4. Airplane don't have enough legroom.	yes	no
5. Bike are better than cars for getting around in a crowded city.	yes	no
6. It's fun to watch bike races like the *Tour de France* on TV.	yes	no
7. Vegetable soups are delicious.	yes	no
8. Fresh vegetable are my favorite food.	yes	no

EXERCISE 35 ▶ Listening and speaking. (Charts 6-1 → 6-9)

Part I. Listen to two friends talking about finding an apartment.

Part II. Complete your own conversation. Perform it for the class. You can use words in the box. NOTE: This conversation is slightly different from Part I.

> Do you know these words?
> - can't afford
> - subway
> - walking distance
> - quiet location
> - dream

air-conditioning	an elevator	near a bus stop	a studio
a balcony	an exercise room	near a freeway	a two-bedroom
close to my job	a laundry room	parking	a walk-up

A: I'm looking for a new place to live.

B: How come?

A: _____. I need _____.

B: I just helped a friend find one. I can help you. What else do you want?

A: I want _____. Also, I _____.

   I don't want _____.

B: Anything else?

A: _____ would be nice.

B: That's expensive.

A: I guess I'm dreaming.

an apartment with a balcony

EXERCISE 36 ▶ Warm-up. (Chart 6-10)

Read the conversation. Look at the personal pronouns in green. Decide if they are subject or object pronouns.

A: Did you hear? Ivan quit his job.
       1

B: I know. I don't understand him. Between you and me, I think it's a bad decision.
   2   3   4   5 6

1. you   subject   object

2. I   subject   object

3. him   subject   object

4. you   subject   object

5. me   subject   object

6. I   subject   object

6-10 Personal Pronouns: Subjects and Objects

SUBJECT PRONOUNS:	*I*	*we*	*you*	*he, she, it*	*they*
OBJECT PRONOUNS:	*me*	*us*	*you*	*him, her, it*	*them*

(a) *Kate* is married. *She* has two children. s	A pronoun refers to a noun. In (a): *she* is a pronoun; it refers to **Kate**. In (b): *her* is a pronoun; it refers to **Kate**. In (a): **She** is a SUBJECT PRONOUN. In (b): **her** is an OBJECT PRONOUN.
(b) *Kate* is my friend. I know *her* well. o	
(c) Mike has *a new blue bike*. He bought *it* yesterday.	A pronoun can refer to a single noun (e.g., **Kate**) or to a noun phrase. In (c): *it* refers to the whole noun phrase *a new blue bike*.
(d) *Eric and I* are good friends. s	Guidelines for using pronouns following *and*: If the pronoun is used as part of the subject, use a subject pronoun, as in (d).
(e) Al met *Eric and me* at the museum. o	If the pronoun is part of the object, use an object pronoun, as in (e) and (f).
(f) Al walked between *Eric and me*. O OF PREP	INCORRECT: *Eric and me are good friends.* INCORRECT: *Al met Eric and I at the museum.*

SINGULAR PRONOUNS:	*I*	*me*	*you*	*he, she, it*	*him, her*
PLURAL PRONOUNS:	*we*	*us*	*you*	*they*	*them*

(g) *Nick* isn't here. *He* is working.	Singular pronouns refer to singular nouns; plural pronouns refer to plural nouns, as in the examples.
(h) The *students* are in class. *They* are taking a test.	
(i) *Kate and Tom* are married. *They* have two children.	

EXERCISE 37 ▸ Looking at grammar. (Chart 6-10)

Write the nouns that the pronouns in green refer to.

1. The desserts looked delicious, but the kids didn't eat them. They are allergic to nuts. They cause breathing problems and itchy skin.

    a. them = _____

    b. They = _____

    c. They = _____

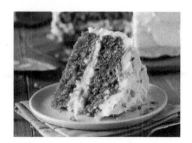 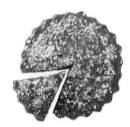 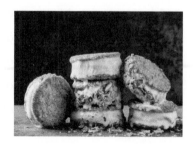

2. Do bees sleep at night? Or do they work in their hives all night long? You never see them after dark. What do they do after night falls?

    a. they = _____

    b. them = _____

    c. they = _____

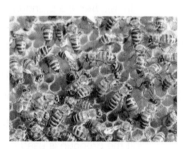

3. Table tennis began in England in the late 1800s. Today it is an international sport. My brother and I played it a lot when we were teenagers. I beat him sometimes, but he was a better player and usually won.

    a. it = _____   c. him = _____

    b. it = _____   d. he = _____

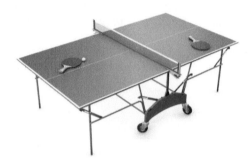

EXERCISE 38 ▶ Looking at grammar. (Chart 6-10)

Circle the correct completions.

1. Toshi ate dinner with   I / me.

2. Toshi ate dinner with Mariko and   I / me.

3. I / me   had dinner with Toshi last night.

4. Toshi drove Mariko and   I / me   to the store after dinner. He waited for   we / us   in the car.

5. We also got tickets for the soccer game. We got   it / them   right away. It / They   is / are   selling fast.

EXERCISE 39 ▶ Looking at grammar. (Chart 6-10)

Complete the sentences with **she, he, it, her, him, they,** or **them**.

1. I have a grammar book. _____*It*_____ is black.

2. Brian borrowed my books. _____ returned _____ yesterday.

3. Sonya is wearing some new earrings. _____ look good on _____.

4. Don't look directly at the sun. Don't look at _____ directly even if you are wearing
   sunglasses. Its light can injure your eyes.

5. Recently, I read about "micromachines." _____ are machines that are smaller
   than a grain of sand. One scientist called _____ "the greatest scientific invention of
   our time."

EXERCISE 40 ▶ Warm-up. (Chart 6-11)

Match each phrase to the picture that it describes.

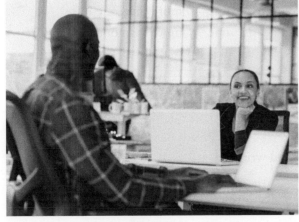

Picture A

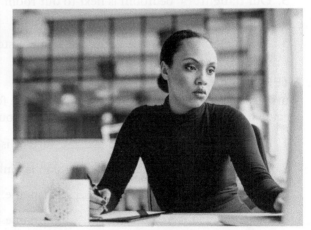

Picture B

1. _____ the teacher's office

2. _____ the teachers' office

6-11 Possessive Nouns

SINGULAR:	(a) I know the *student's* name.	An apostrophe (') and an **-s** are used with nouns to show possession.
PLURAL:	(b) I know the *students'* names.	
PLURAL:	(c) I know the *children's* names.	

SINGULAR	(d) the student → the *student's* name my baby → my *baby's* name a man → a *man's* name		**SINGULAR POSSESSIVE NOUN:** *noun + apostrophe (') + -s*
	(e) James → *James'/James's* name		A singular noun that ends in **-s** has two possible possessive forms: *James'* or *James's*.
PLURAL	(f) the students → the *students'* names my babies → my *babies'* names		**PLURAL POSSESSIVE NOUN:** *noun + -s + apostrophe (')*
	(g) men → *men's* names the children → the *children's* names		**IRREGULAR PLURAL POSSESSIVE NOUN:** *noun + apostrophe (') + -s* (An irregular plural noun is a plural noun that does not end in **-s**: *children, men, people, women*. See Chart 6-1.)
COMPARE: (h) *Tom's* here. (i) *Tom's* brother is here.			In (h): **Tom's** is not a possessive noun. It is a contraction of *Tom is*, used in informal writing. In (i): **Tom's** is a possessive noun.

EXERCISE 41 ▶ Looking at grammar. (Chart 6-11)
Decide if the meaning of the word in green is "one" or "more than one."

1. The teacher answered the student's questions.   (one)   more than one
2. The teacher answered the students' questions.   one   more than one
3. Our daughters' bedroom is next to our room.   one   more than one
4. Our son's room is downstairs.   one   more than one
5. Men's clothing is on sale at the department store.   one   more than one

EXERCISE 42 ▶ Game: trivia. (Chart 6-11)
Work in small groups. Use the correct possessive form of each noun to complete the sentences. Decide if the information is true or false. The group with the most correct answers wins.★

1. *earth*   The _____ surface is about 70% water.   T   F
2. *elephant*   An _____ skin is pink and wrinkled.   T   F
3. *man*   Pat is a _____ name.   T   F
4. *woman*   Pat is a _____ name.   T   F
5. *women*   The area for language is larger in _____ brains.   T   F
6. *person*   A _____ eyes blink more if he/she is nervous.   T   F
7. *People*   _____ voices always get lower as they age.   T   F

★See *Trivia Answers*, p. 247.

EXERCISE 43 ▸ Grammar and speaking. (Chart 6-11)

Part I. Look at the Nelson family tree. Complete the sentences using the correct possessive form.

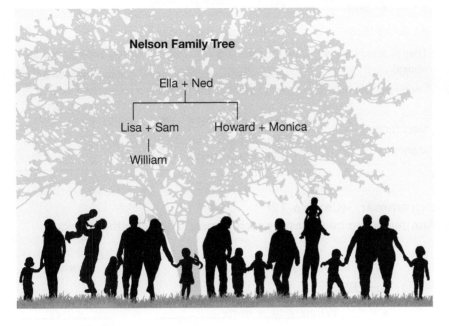

Nelson Family Tree

Ella + Ned

Lisa + Sam   Howard + Monica

William

1. _____Ned's_____ wife is Ella.

2. _____ husband is Sam.

3. Howard is _____ brother.

4. Howard is _____ husband.

5. _____ grandmother is Ella.

6. _____ parents are Sam and Lisa.

7. Ella and _____ grandson is William.

8. Howard and Monica are _____ aunt and uncle.

Part II. Work with a partner. Talk about the members of your family or another family. Use possessives. Your partner will create a family tree from your description.

EXERCISE 44 ▸ Warm-up. (Chart 6-12)

Choose the correct answers.

1. Who's holding the little girl in the striped shirt?
   a. That's Rachel.   b. That's Rachel's.

2. Whose granddaughter is that?
   a. That's Rachel.   b. That's Rachel's.

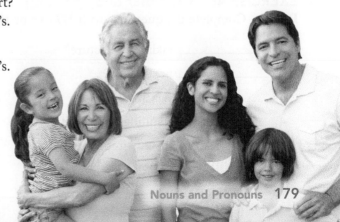

6-12 Using *Whose*

Question	Answer	
(a) *Whose (book)* is this?	It's John's (book).	*Whose* asks about possession.
(b) *Whose (books)* are those?	They're mine (OR my books).	The meaning in (a): *Who does this book belong to?*
(c) *Whose car* did you borrow?	I borrowed Karen's (car).	NOTE: The person asking the question may omit the noun (*book*) if the meaning is clear to the listener.
COMPARE: (d) *Who's* that? (e) *Whose* is that?	Mary Smith. Mary's.	*Who's* and *whose* have the same pronunciation. *Who's* is a contraction of *who is*. *Whose* asks about possession.

EXERCISE 45 ▸ Looking at grammar. (Chart 6-12)
Using *who's* or *whose* with *that*, make two questions for each picture. Then give the correct answer for each question.

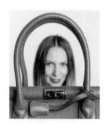

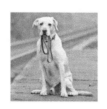

	QUESTION	ANSWER
1. *bag / Elise*		
a.	Whose bag is that?	Elise's
b.	Who's that?	Elise
2. *Jason / apple*		
a.	_____	_____
b.	_____	_____
3. *car / Roger*		
a.	_____	_____
b.	_____	_____
4. *Buddy / leash*		
a.	_____	_____
b.	_____	_____

EXERCISE 46 ▸ Grammar and speaking. (Chart 6-12)
Part I. Complete the questions with *Whose* or *Who's*.

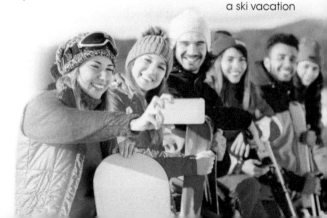
a ski vacation

1. _____ taking the picture?
2. _____ next to you?
3. _____ skis are those?
4. _____ standing at the end?
5. _____ the guy in the hat?

6. _____ house did you stay at?

Part II. Ask another student two additional questions, one with **Who's** and one with **Whose**.

EXERCISE 47 ▶ Listening. (Chart 6-12)
Listen to the each question and choose the correct word.

1. Who's   Whose   3. Who's   Whose   5. Who's   Whose

2. Who's   Whose   4. Who's   Whose   6. Who's   Whose

EXERCISE 48 ▶ Warm-up. (Chart 6-13)
Check (✓) all the grammatically correct responses.

Do you know whose camera this is?

1. _____ It's my camera.   4. _____ It's yours.   7. _____ It's theirs.

2. _____ It's mine.   5. _____ It's your camera. 8. _____ It's their camera.

3. _____ It's my.   6. _____ It's your's.   9. _____ It's theirs'.

6-13	Possessive Pronouns and Adjectives	

This pen belongs to me.		Examples (a) and (b) have the same meaning; they both show possession.
(a) It's *mine*.		
(b) It is *my* pen.		*Mine* is a *possessive pronoun; **my*** is a *possessive adjective.*

Possessive Pronouns	**Possessive Adjectives**	A POSSESSIVE PRONOUN is used alone, without a noun following it.
(c) I have *mine*.	I have *my* pen.	A POSSESSIVE ADJECTIVE is used only with a noun following it.
(d) You have *yours*.	You have *your* pen.	
(e) She has *hers*.	She has *her* pen.	INCORRECT: *I have mine pen.*
(f) He has *his*.	He has *his* pen.	INCORRECT: *I have my.*
(g) We have *ours*.	We have *our* pens.	
(h) You have *yours*.	You have *your* pens.	
(i) They have *theirs*.	They have *their* pens.	
(j) ————	I have a book.	
	Its cover is black.	

COMPARE *its* vs. *it's*:	In (k): *its* (NO apostrophe) is a possessive adjective modifying the noun *name*.
(k) Jon gave me a book. I don't remember *its* name.	
(l) Jon gave me a book. *It's* really interesting.	In (l): *It's* (with an apostrophe) is a contraction of *it + is*.

COMPARE *their* vs. *there* vs. *they're*:	***Their, there***, and ***they're*** have the same pronunciation, but not the same meaning.
(m) The students have *their* books.	***their*** = possessive adjective, as in (m)
(n) My books are over *there*.	***there*** = an expression of place, as in (n)
(o) Where are the students? *They're* in class.	***they're*** = *they are,* as in (o)

EXERCISE 49 ▸ Looking at grammar. (Chart 6-13)
Circle the correct completions.

1. Alice called (her) / hers   friend.

2. Hasan wrote a letter to   his / he's   mother.

3. It's / Its   normal for a dog to chase   it's / its   tail.

4. The cat cleaned   its / it's   fur with   its / it's   tongue.

5. Paula drove my car to work.   Hers / Her   had a flat tire.

6. Junko fell off her bike and broke   hers / her   arm.

7. Anastasia is a good friend of   my / mine.*

8. I met a friend of   you / yours   yesterday.

9. A: Excuse me. Is this   my / mine   pen or   your / yours?

   B: This one is   my / mine.   Your / Yours   is on   your / yours   desk.

10. a. Adam and Amanda are married.   They / They're   live in an apartment building.

    b. Their / There / They're   apartment is on the fifth floor.

    c. We live in the same building.   Our / Ours   apartment has one bedroom, but
       their / theirs   has two.

    d. Their / There / They're   sitting   their / there / they're   now because
       their / there / they're   waiting for a visit from   their / there / they're son.

EXERCISE 50 ▸ Let's talk. (Charts 6-12 and 6-13)
Work in small groups. Take pictures of objects in the room (about 10-15 per
group) with cell phones. Ask and answer questions about the objects. Use
possessive pronouns, possessive adjectives, or the person's name.

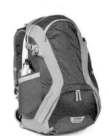

Example: (picture of a backpack)
STUDENT A: Whose backpack is this?
STUDENT B: It's hers. / It's her backpack. / It's Yumi's.

EXERCISE 51 ▸ Warm-up. (Chart 6-14)
Work in small groups. Take turns saying the sentences while you or other students show the
meaning with a small mirror.

1. I am looking at myself.
2. You are looking at yourself.
3. You are looking at yourselves.
4. He is looking at himself.
5. They are looking at themselves.
6. She is looking at herself.
7. We are looking at ourselves.

---

*A friend of + possessive pronoun (e.g., a *friend of mine*) is a common expression.

6-14 Reflexive Pronouns

myself	(a) *I saw myself in the mirror.*	REFLEXIVE PRONOUNS end in **-self/-selves**. They are used when the subject (e.g., *I*) and the object (e.g., *myself*) are the same person.
yourself	(b) *You (one person) saw yourself.*	
herself	(c) *She saw herself.*	
himself	(d) *He saw himself.*	INCORRECT: *I saw me in the mirror.*
itself	(e) *It (e.g., the kitten) saw itself.*	
ourselves	(f) *We saw ourselves.*	
yourselves	(g) *You (plural) saw yourselves.*	
themselves	(h) *They saw themselves.*	

(i) *Greg lives by himself.*	**By** + a reflexive pronoun = alone
(j) *I sat by myself on the park bench.*	In (i): Greg lives alone, without family or roommates.
(k) *I enjoyed myself at the fair.*	*Enjoy* and a few other verbs are commonly followed by a reflexive pronoun. See the list below.

Common Expressions with Reflexive Pronouns

believe in yourself	feel sorry for yourself	pinch yourself	tell yourself
blame yourself	give yourself (something)	be proud of yourself	work for yourself
cut yourself	help yourself	take care of yourself	wish yourself (luck)
drive yourself	hurt yourself	talk to yourself	
enjoy yourself	introduce yourself	teach yourself	

EXERCISE 52 ▸ Looking at grammar. (Chart 6-14)

Complete the sentences with reflexive pronouns.

1. Are you OK, Heidi? Did you hurt ____*yourself*____?

2. Leo taught _____ to play the piano. He never had a teacher.

3. Do you ever talk to _____? Most people talk to _____ sometimes.

4. A newborn baby can't take care of _____.

5. We need to have confidence in our own abilities. We need to believe in _____.

6. Isabel always wishes _____ good luck before a big test.

7. Kazu, there's plenty of food on the table. Please help _____.

8. I couldn't believe my luck! I had to pinch _____ to make sure I wasn't dreaming.

EXERCISE 53 ▶ Let's talk: interview. (Chart 6-14)

Interview six students. Ask each student a different question. Share some of their answers.

1. In this town, what is a good way to enjoy yourself?
2. How do people introduce themselves in your country? What do they say?
3. Have you ever wished yourself good luck? When or why?
4. Have you ever felt sorry for yourself? Or, have you ever felt proud of yourself? If so, why?
5. When athletes talk to themselves before an important event, what do you imagine they say?
6. In your country, at what age does a person usually begin living by himself or herself?

EXERCISE 54 ▶ Warm-up. (Chart 6-15)

Choose the picture that matches the description: *One flower is red. Another is yellow. The other is pink.*

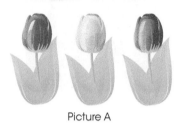

Picture A

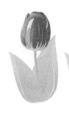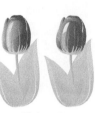

Picture B

6-15	Singular Forms of *Other: Another* vs. *The Other*

Another

one another ○ ○ ○	**another** = one more out of a group of items ***Another*** is a combination of *an + other*, written as one word.
(a) Paul is looking at baseball caps. The store has several that he likes. One is blue. *Another* is red.	

The Other

one the other	**the other** = all that remains of a given number; the last one
(b) Paul is looking at baseball caps in the store. There are two colors. One is blue. *The other* is red.	

| (c) Paul tried on one cap. Then he tried on { *another cap.* / *another one.* / *another.* | ***Another*** and ***the other*** can be used

• as adjectives in front of a noun (e.g., ***another cap***).
• as adjectives in front of the word ***one*** (e.g., ***another one***).
• alone as pronouns (e.g., ***another***). |
| (d) Paul tried on one cap. Then he tried on { *the other cap.* / *the other one.* / *the other.* | |

EXERCISE 55 ▶ Looking at grammar. (Chart 6-15)
Complete the sentences with *another* or *the other*.

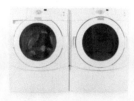

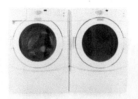

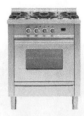

Picture A   Picture B

1. One appliance in Picture A is a washing machine. _____ is a dryer.

2. There are three appliances in Picture B. One is a washing machine. Another is a dryer.

   _____ is a stove.

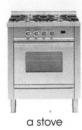   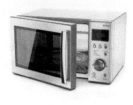   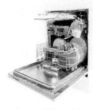   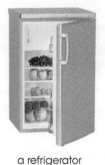

a stove   a microwave   a dishwasher   a refrigerator

3. There are many, many types of appliances. One is a stove.

   a. _____ is a microwave.

   b. _____ is a dishwasher.

   c. What is the name of _____ type of appliance?

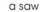   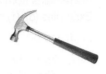

a saw   a hammer   a screwdriver   a wrench

4. Do you know the names of these tools? One is a saw. _____ is a hammer.

5. I need to borrow two tools. One is a screwdriver. _____ is a hammer.

6. Here are four tools. One is a saw. _____ is a hammer.

   _____ is a screwdriver. _____ is a wrench.

7. A builder needs many, many tools. One is a saw. _____ is a hammer.

   _____ is a screwdriver. _____ is a wrench.

EXERCISE 56 ▸ Warm-up. (Chart 6-16)
Match the sentences to the correct pictures.

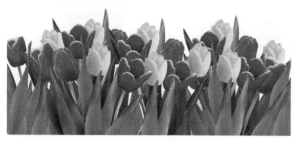

Picture A

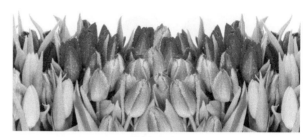

Picture B

1. _____ Some are red. The others are yellow.

2. _____ Some are red. Others are yellow.

6-16 Plural Forms of *Other*: *Other(s)* vs. *The Other(s)*

Other(s)

some   other(s)

Jeremy has many kinds of fruit trees in his garden. Some have apples.

(a) *Other trees* have peaches.

(b) *Other ones* have peaches.

(c) *Others have* peaches.

Other(s) (without *the*) means "several more out of a group of similar items, several in addition to the one(s) already mentioned." Examples (a)–(c) have the same meaning.

In (a) and (b): *Other* is an adjective.

In (c): *Others* is a pronoun.
   Others = *Other trees*

INCORRECT: *Others ones*
       Others trees

The Other(s)

some   the other(s)

Lara has two kinds of fruit trees in her garden. Some have pears.

(d) *The other trees* have cherries.

(e) *The other ones* have cherries.

(f) *The others* have cherries.

The other(s) means "the last ones in a specific group, the remains from a given number of similar items." Examples (d)–(f) have the same meaning.

In (d) and (e): *The other* is an adjective.

In (f): *The others* is a pronoun.
   The others = *The other trees*

INCORRECT: *The others ones*
       The others trees

EXERCISE 57 ▸ Grammar and speaking. (Charts 6-15 and 6-16)
Work in pairs or small groups. Perform these actions.

1. Hold two pens. Use a form of *other* to describe the second pen.
    → *I'm holding two pens. One is mine, and the other belongs to Ahmed.*

2. Hold three pens. Use a form of *other* to describe the second and third pens.

3. Hold up your two hands. One of them is your right hand. Tell us about your left hand, using a form of *other*.

4. Hold up your right hand. One of the five fingers is your thumb. Using forms of *other*, tell us about your index finger, then your middle finger, then your ring finger, and then your little finger, the last of the five fingers on your right hand.

EXERCISE 58 ▸ Looking at grammar. (Chart 6-16)
Complete the sentences with *other*, *others*, *the other*, or *the others*.

1. There are many kinds of animals in the world. The elephant is one kind. Some ____*others*____ are tigers, horses, and bears.

2. There are many kinds of animals in the world. The elephant is one kind. Some _____ kinds are tigers, horses, and bears.

3. There are three colors in the Italian flag. One of the colors is red. _____ are green and white.

4. There are three colors in the Italian flag. One of the colors is red. _____ colors are green and white.

5. Many people like to get up very early in the morning. _____ like to sleep until noon.

6. There are many kinds of geometric shapes. Some are circles. _____ shapes are squares. Still _____ are rectangles.

7. There are four geometric shapes in the above drawing. One is a square. _____ shapes are a rectangle, a circle, and a triangle.

8. Of the four geometric shapes in the drawing, only the circle has curved lines. _____ have straight lines.

6-17 Summary: Forms of *Other*

	Adjective	Pronoun	
SINGULAR	another apple	another	Note that the word ***others*** (***other*** + *final* **-s**) is used only as a plural pronoun.
PLURAL	other apples	other**s**	
SINGULAR	the other apple	the other	
PLURAL	the other apples	the other**s**	

EXERCISE 59 ▸ Looking at grammar. (Chart 6-17)
Look at each picture and complete the sentences with the words in the box.

another	other	others	the other	the others

1. There is a large bowl of apples on the table. Paul ate one apple. He is still hungry. He wants a second one.

   a. He wants to eat _____ apple.

   b. He wants to eat _____ one.

   c. He wants to eat _____ .

   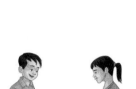

2. There are two apples on the table. Paul is going to eat one of them.

   a. Sara is going to eat _____ apple.

   b. Sara is going to eat _____ one.

   c. Sara is going to eat _____ .

3. There are many apples in Paul's kitchen. Paul is holding one apple.

   a. There are _____ apples in a bowl.

   b. There are _____ ones on a plate.

   c. There are _____ on a chair.

   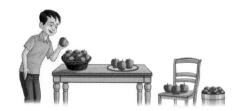

4. There are four apples on the table. Paul is going to take one of them, and Sara is going to take three.

   a. Sara is going to take _____ apples.

   b. Sara is going to take _____ ones.

   c. Sara is going to take _____ .

   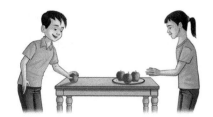

EXERCISE 60 ▶ Looking at grammar. (Charts 6-15 → 6-17)
Complete the sentences with *another*, *other*, *others*, *the other*, or *the others*.

1. Juan doesn't like to wear suits. He has only one. His wife wants him to buy _____ _another_ _____ one.

2. Juan is looking at two suits. One is blue, and _____ is brown.

3. Some suits are blue. _____ are gray.

4. Some jackets have zippers. _____ jackets have buttons.

5. Some people keep dogs as pets. _____ have cats. Still _____ people have fish or birds as pets.

6. My boyfriend gave me a ring. I tried to put it on my ring finger, but it didn't fit. So I had to put it on _____ finger.

7. People have two thumbs. One is on the right hand. _____ is on the left hand.

8. Sometimes when I'm thirsty, I'll have a glass of water, but often one glass isn't enough, so I'll have _____ one.

9. There are five letters in the word *fresh*. One of the letters is a vowel. _____ are consonants.

10. Smith is a common last name in English. _____ common names are Johnson, Jones, Miller, Anderson, Moore, and Brown.

EXERCISE 61 ▶ Looking at grammar. (Charts 6-15 → 6-17)
Read each conversation and choose the correct statement (a. or b.).

1. A: Did you buy the black jacket?
   B: No. I bought the other one.

   a. Speaker B was looking at two jackets.
   b. Speaker B was looking at several jackets.

2. A: One of my favorite colors is dark blue. Another one is red.
   B: Me too.

   a. The speakers have only two favorite colors.
   b. The speakers have more than two favorite colors.

3. A: Do your friends live on campus?
   B: A few live on campus, and the others live nearby.

   a. All of Speaker B's friends live on or near campus.
   b. Some of Speaker B's friends live on or near campus.

4. A: This looks like the wrong street. Let's go back and take the other road.

   B: OK.

   a. There are several roads the speakers can take.

   b. There are two roads the speakers can take.

5. A: What's the best way to get downtown from here?

   B: It's pretty far to walk. Some people take the bus. Others prefer the subway.

   a. There are only two ways to get downtown.

   b. There are more than two ways to get downtown.

6. A: When I was a kid, I had lots of pets. One was a black dog. Another was an orange cat.
      Some others were a goldfish and a turtle.

   B: Pets are great for kids.

   a. Speaker A had more than four pets.

   b. Speaker A had only four pets.

7. A: I'm packing a banana for my lunch. Do you want the other?

   B: Sure, thanks.

   a. There are two bananas.

   b. There are several bananas.

EXERCISE 62 ▸ Check your knowledge. (Chapter 6 Review)

Correct the errors.

1. Jimmy had three *wishes* ~~wish~~ for his birthday.

2. I had some black beans soup for lunch.

3. The windows in our classroom is dirty.

4. People in Brazil speaks Portuguese.

5. Are around 8,600 types of birds in the world.

6. My mother and father work in Milan. Their teacher's.

7. In my family, mens and womens work as carpenter, pilot, and doctor.

8. Is a new student in our class. Have you met her?

9. There are two pool at the park. The smaller one is for childs. The another is for adults.

10. The highways in my country are excellents.

11. I don't like my apartment. Its in a bad neighborhood. Is a lot of crime. I'm going to move to

    other neighborhood.

EXERCISE 63 ▸ Reading and writing. (Chapter 6)

Part I. Read the passage and answer the questions.

Do you know these words?
- calm   - techniques
- nervous   - wave
- anxious   - inhale/exhale
- variety   - heart rate

HOW TO CALM YOURSELF

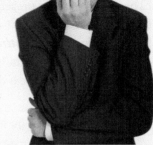

Everyone feels nervous or anxious at times. Maybe it comes from an experience like going to the dentist. Or perhaps it's worrying about a big test. There are a variety of techniques that people use to calm themselves. Here are three that many people have found helpful.

One way to relax is by imagining a peaceful place, such as a tropical beach. Thinking about the warm water, cool breezes, and regular sounds of the ocean waves helps people calm themselves. Another popular method is deep breathing. A person inhales deeply and then slowly exhales as a way to slow the heart rate and relax the body. Still other people find exercise helpful. Some people benefit from a slow activity like a 20-minute walk. Others prefer activities that make them tired, like running or swimming.

After people try some of these techniques, many feel better just knowing that they can use their mind or physical exercise to help them relax.

1. What are three ways people relax when they are nervous? (Use **one** and **another** in your answer.)
2. Why do some people choose activities like running and swimming as a way to relax?
3. Imagine you are trying to relax by thinking of a peaceful place. What place would you think of?
4. How do you relax when you are nervous?

Part II. Read this paragraph by a student who tells how he relaxes when he's nervous.

How I Calm Down

Sometimes I feel nervous, especially when I have to give a speech. My body begins to shake, and I realize that I have to calm myself down. This is the technique I use: I imagine myself in a peaceful place. My favorite place in the world is the sea. I imagine myself on the water. I am floating. I feel the warm water around me. The sounds around me are very relaxing. I only hear the waves and maybe a few birds. I don't think about the past or the future. I can feel my heart rate decrease a little, and my body slowly starts to calm down. Before I give a speech, I use this technique. I find it very helpful.

Part III. Write a paragraph about how you relax when you are nervous. Follow the model in Part II. Give specific details about how you relax and what the results are.

Sometimes I feel nervous, especially when I have to _____. My

_____ and I realize that I have to calm myself down. This is the technique

I use: _____.

WRITING TIP

When you want to add interesting details to your writing, it is helpful to ask yourself these questions: *who, what, when, where, why,* and *how.* For this writing assignment, it can help you think of details to describe how you calm yourself. For example, what do you do, exactly, to calm yourself? Where are you? What do you see? How do you feel? Why do you feel better?

Part IV. Edit your writing. Check for the following:

1. ☐ use of the simple present to describe your feelings and actions
2. ☐ correct use of final *-s*/*-es*/*-ies* on singular verbs
3. ☐ correct forms of ***another***/***other*** if you use these words
4. ☐ use of interesting details in your paragraph
5. ☐ correct spelling (use a dictionary or spell-check)

▨▨▪▪■ For digital resources, go to the Pearson Practice English app.

Modal Auxiliaries, the Imperative, Making Suggestions, Stating Preferences

PRETEST: What do I already know?

Write "C" if the **boldfaced** words are correct and "I" if they are incorrect.

1. _____ We **have to wake** up early tomorrow. Our flight leaves at 5:00. (Chart 7-1)

2. _____ I **can read** when I was four years old. (Chart 7-2)

3. _____ The weather **might** hot this weekend. (Chart 7-3)

4. _____ Ben isn't here. He **could** still **be** asleep. (Chart 7-4)

5. _____ **May** I please **go** to a movie tonight? (Chart 7-5)

6. _____ **May** you **go** with me to the mall? (Chart 7-6)

7. _____ **Maybe** I **should** wear a warm coat. It's pretty cold outside. (Chart 7-7)

8. _____ **You better get** ready. We're going to be late. (Chart 7-8)

9. _____ I**'ve got to leave**. I need to pick up my kids at school. (Chart 7-9)

10. _____ I **must not study** this weekend. Our teacher didn't give us any homework. (Chart 7-10)

11. _____ There is only one room available at the hotel. It **must be** popular. (Chart 7-11)

12. _____ The information **could be** clearer, couldn't it? (Chart 7-12)

13. _____ Please **don't to wear** your shoes indoors. (Chart 7-13)

14. _____ It's a nice evening. Why **we don't eat** dinner outside on the patio? (Chart 7-14)

15. _____ My parents **would rather living** in a small town than a large city. (Chart 7-15)

EXERCISE 1 ▶ Warm-up. (Chart 7-1)

Check (✓) the sentences that are grammatically correct.

1. _____ I can skydive.

2. _____ He cans skydives.

3. _____ She can to skydive.

4. _____ My parents can't skydive.

7-1 Introduction to Modal Auxiliaries

The verbs in this chapter are called "modal auxiliaries." They are helping verbs that express a wide range of meanings such as ability, possibility, and necessity.*

Auxiliary + the Simple Form of a Verb

can	(a) Olga *can speak* English.	Some modal auxiliaries are immediately followed by the simple form of a verb, as in (a)–(e).
could	(b) He *couldn't come* to class.	
may	(c) It *may rain* tomorrow.	• They are not followed by *to*.
will	(d) I *will be* in class tomorrow.	INCORRECT: *Olga can to speak English.*
would	(e) *Would* you please *close* the door?	• The main verb does not have a final *-s*.
		INCORRECT: *Olga can speaks English.*
		• The main verb is not in a past form.
		INCORRECT: *Olga can spoke English.*
		• The main verb is not in its *-ing* form.
		INCORRECT: *Olga can speaking English.*

Auxiliary + *to* + the Simple Form of a Verb

have to	(f) I *have to study* tonight.	Some modal auxiliaries use *to* + the simple form, as in (f) and (g).
be able to	(g) Kate *is able to learn* quickly.	

*See Chart 7-16 for a summary of all the modal auxiliaries in this chapter.

EXERCISE 2 ▸ Looking at grammar. (Chart 7-1)
Make sentences with the given verbs + *come*. Add *to* where necessary. Follow the example.

Example: can → *Leo can come tonight.*

1. may
2. is able
3. has
4. will not
5. could not
6. is not able

EXERCISE 3 ▸ Listening. (Chart 7-1)
Listen to the sentences. Add *to* where necessary. If *to* isn't necessary, write **Ø**. Notice that *to* may sound like "ta."

Plans for Tomorrow

A: Where do you and Joe have ___1___ go tomorrow?

B: I have ___2___ go downtown. Joe has ___3___ take the kids to buy school supplies. He couldn't ___4___ do it today.

A: May I ___5___ come with you?

B: You can ___6___ if you want to get up early.

A: Would you ___7___ wake me up? Sometimes I'm not able ___8___ hear my alarm.

B: Sure. I have a great way to wake people up. You definitely won't ___9___ sleep in!

A: I can't ___10___ wait!

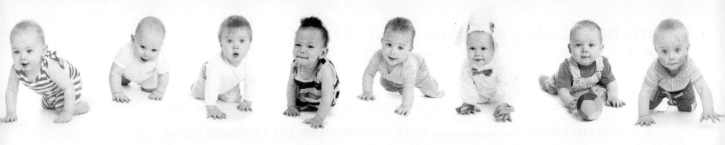

EXERCISE 4 ▶ Warm-up. (Chart 7-2)

Circle a completion for each sentence. Answers may vary. Discuss your answers.

1. A newborn baby   can / can't   roll over.

2. A baby of four months   can / can't   smile.

3. A newborn baby   is able to / isn't able to   see black and white shapes.

4. A baby of six months   is able to / isn't able to   see colors.

5. When I was nine months old, I   could / couldn't   crawl.

6. When I was nine months old, I   could / couldn't   walk.

7-2 Expressing Ability: *Can, Could, Be Able To*	
(a) Bob *can play* the piano. (b) You *can buy* a screwdriver at a hardware store. (c) I *can meet* you at Ted's tomorrow afternoon.	*Can* expresses *ability* in the present or future.
(d) I $\begin{cases} can't \\ cannot \\ can\ not \end{cases}$ understand that sentence.	The negative form of *can* may be written *can't*, *cannot*, or *can not*.
(e) I *can gó*. (f) I *cán't* go.	In spoken English, *can* is usually unstressed and pronounced /kən/ = "kun." *Can't* is stressed and pronounced /kæn?/, with the final sound being a glottal stop.* The glottal stop replaces the /t/ in spoken English. Occasionally native speakers have trouble hearing the difference between *can* and *can't* and need to ask for clarification.
(g) Our son *could walk* when he was one year old.	The past form of *can* is *could*.
(h) He *couldn't walk* when he was six months old.	The negative of *could* is *couldn't* or *could not*.
(i) He *can read*. (j) He *is able to read*. (k) She *could read*. (l) She *was able to read*.	Ability can also be expressed with a form of *be able to*. Examples (i) and (j) have the same meaning. Examples (k) and (l) have the same meaning.

*A glottal stop is the sound you hear in the negative "unh-uh." The air is stopped by the closing of your glottis in the back of your throat. The phonetic symbol for the glottal stop is /?/.

EXERCISE 5 ▸ Looking at grammar. (Chart 7-2)

Part I. Complete the sentences with **can** or **can't**.

1. A dog _____ swim, but it _____ fly.

2. A frog _____ live both on land and in water, but a cat _____ .

3. A bilingual person _____ speak three languages, but a trilingual person

   _____ .

4. Many people with color blindness _____ see green and red, but people with normal

   color vision _____ .

Part II. Restate the sentences in Part I. Use **be able to**.

EXERCISE 6 ▸ Let's talk: interview. (Chart 7-2)

Interview your classmates. Ask each student a different question. If the answer is "yes," ask the follow-up question in parentheses. Share some of your answers with the class.

Can you …

1. speak more than two languages? (Which ones?)
2. draw well — for example, draw a picture of me? (Can you do it now?)
3. fold a piece of paper in half more than six times? (Can you show me?)
4. play chess? (How long have you played?)

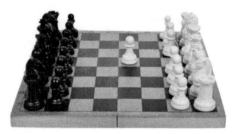

Are you able to …

5. write clearly with both your right and left hands? (Can you show me?)
6. pat the top of your head with one hand and rub your stomach in a circle with the other hand at the same time? (Can you show me?)
7. hold your breath underwater for a long time? (How long?)
8. play a musical instrument? (Which one?)

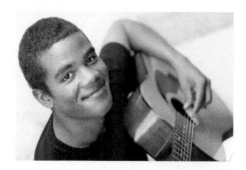

Listen to the conversation. You will hear reductions for **can** and **can't**. Write the words you hear.

In the Classroom

A: I _____ this math assignment.
            ₁

B: I _____ you with that.
      ₂

A: Really? _____ this problem to me?
          ₃

B: Well, we _____ out the answer until we do this part.
        ₄

A: OK. But it's so hard.

B: Yeah, but I know you _____ it. Just go slowly.
                ₅

A: I need to leave in a few minutes. _____ me after school today to finish this?
                                        ₆

B: Well, I _____ you right after school, but how about at 5:00?
        ₇

A: Great!

Complete the sentences with **could/couldn't/be able to/not be able to** and your own words.

Example: A year ago I ____ , but now I can. → *A year ago I couldn't speak English, but now I can.*

1. When I was a child, I ____ , but now I can.
2. When I was six, I ____ , but I wasn't able to do that when I was three.
3. I ____ when I was younger, but now I can't.
4. In the past, I ____ , but now I am.

Check (✓) the sentences in each group that have the same meaning.

GROUP A

1. ____ Maybe it will be hot tomorrow.

2. ____ It might be hot tomorrow.

3. ____ It may be hot tomorrow.

GROUP B

4. ____ You can have dessert now.

5. ____ You may have dessert now.

GROUP C

6. ____ She can't stay up late.

7. ____ She might not stay up late.

7-3 Expressing Possibility: *May, Might,* and *Maybe;* Expressing Permission: *May* and *Can*

(a) It *may rain* tomorrow. (b) It *might rain* tomorrow. (c) — Why isn't John in class? — I don't know. He $\left\{\begin{array}{l}may\\might\end{array}\right\}$ be sick today.	***May*** and ***might*** express possibility in the present or future. They have the same meaning. There is no difference in meaning between (a) and (b).
(d) It *may not rain* tomorrow. (e) It *might not rain* tomorrow.	Negative: ***may not*** and ***might not*** (Do not contract ***may*** and ***might*** with ***not***.)
(f) *Maybe* it will rain tomorrow. COMPARE: (g) *Maybe* John is sick. (adverb) (h) John *may be* sick. (verb)	In (f) and (g): ***maybe*** (spelled as one word) is an adverb. It means "possibly." It comes at the beginning of a sentence. INCORRECT: *It will maybe rain tomorrow.* In (h): ***may be*** (two words) is a verb form: the modal ***may*** + the main verb ***be***. Examples (g) and (h) have the same meaning. INCORRECT: *John maybe sick.*
(i) Passengers with young children *may board* now. (j) Passengers with young children *can board* now.	***May*** is also used to give *permission*, as in (i). ***Can*** is often used to give *permission*, too, as in (j). NOTE: Examples (i) and (j) have the same meaning, but ***may*** is more formal than ***can***.
(k) You *may not have* a cookie. You *can't have* a cookie.	***May not*** and ***cannot*** (***can't***) are used to deny permission (i.e., to say "no").

EXERCISE 10 ▶ Looking at grammar. (Chart 7-3)
Rewrite the sentences with the words in parentheses.

1. It may snow tonight.

   (*might*) _____

   (*Maybe*) _____

2. You might need to wear your boots.

   (*may*) _____

   (*Maybe*) _____

   _____

3. Maybe there will be a blizzard.

   (*may*) _____

   (*might*) _____

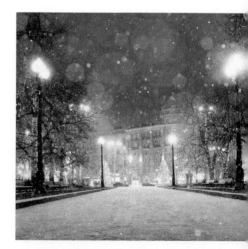

EXERCISE 11 ▶ Let's talk. (Chart 7-3)

Answer each question with **may**, **might**, and **maybe**. Include at least three possibilities in each answer. Work in pairs, in small groups, or as a class.

Example: What are you going to do tomorrow?
→ *I don't know.* ***I may*** *go downtown.* OR ***I might*** *go to the laundromat.*
Maybe *I'll study all day. Who knows?*

1. What are you going to do tomorrow night?
2. What's the weather going to be like tomorrow?
3. What is our teacher going to do tonight?
4. (_____) isn't in class today. Where is he/she?
5. What is your occupation going to be ten years from now?

EXERCISE 12 ▶ Looking at grammar. (Chart 7-3)

Complete the sentences with **can**, **may**, or **might**. Identify the meaning of the modals: possibility or permission.

In a Courtroom

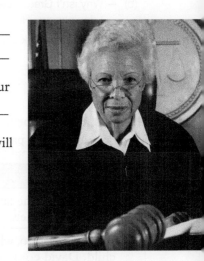

1. No one speaks without the judge's permission. You _____*may / can*_____ not speak until the judge asks you a question. *Meaning:* _____*permission*_____

2. The judge _____ or _____ not reduce your fine for your speeding ticket. It depends. Meaning: _____

3. You _____ not argue with the judge. If you argue, you will get a fine. Meaning: _____

4. You have a strong case, but I'm not sure if you will convince the judge. You _____ win or you _____ lose.
Meaning: _____

EXERCISE 13 ▶ Listening. (Charts 7-2 and 7-3)

You will hear sentences with **can**, **may**, or **might**. Decide if the speakers are expressing ability, possibility, or permission.

Example: You will hear: A: Where's Victor?
                                        B: I don't know. He may be sick.

        You will choose: ability   (possibility)   permission

1. ability   possibility   permission
2. ability   possibility   permission
3. ability   possibility   permission
4. ability   possibility   permission
5. ability   possibility   permission

EXERCISE 14. Warm-up. (Chart 7-4)

In which sentence is the speaker expressing the following?

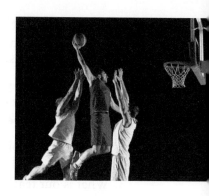

a. past ability   b. present possibility   c. future possibility

1. _____ The score is 80–90, but with five minutes left, our team could win.

2. _____ A player is on the ground. He could be hurt.

3. _____ Our team didn't win. We couldn't score another basket.

7-4 Using *Could* to Express Possibility

(a) — How was the movie? *Could* you *understand* the English? — Not very well. I *could* only *understand* it with the help of subtitles.	One meaning of **could** is *past ability,* as in (a).* Another meaning of **could** is *possibility*.
(b) — Why isn't Greg in class? — I don't know. He *could be* sick.	In (b): **He could be sick** has the same meaning as *He may/might be sick,* i.e., *It is possible that he is sick.* In (b): **could** expresses a *present* possibility.
(c) Look at those dark clouds. It *could rain* any minute.	In (c): **could** expresses a *future* possibility.

*See also Chart 7-2.

EXERCISE 15 ▶ Looking at grammar. (Charts 7-2 and 7-4)

Does **could** express past, present, or future time? What is the meaning: ability or possibility?

SENTENCE	PAST	PRESENT	FUTURE	ABILITY	POSSIBILITY
1. I could be home late tonight. Don't wait for me for dinner.			X		X
2. Thirty years ago, when he was a small child, David could speak Swahili fluently. Now he's forgotten a lot of it.					
3. A: Where's Alicia? B: I don't know. She could be at the mall.					
4. When I was a child, I could climb trees, but now I'm too old.					
5. Let's leave for the airport now. Yuki's plane could arrive early, and we want to be there when she arrives.					
6. A: What's that on the carpet? B: I don't know. It looks like a bug. Or it could be a piece of fuzz.					

EXERCISE 16 ▸ Let's talk. (Chart 7-4)

Suggest possible solutions for each situation. Use *could*. Work in pairs, in small groups, or as a class.

Finding Solutions

Example: Tim has to go to work early tomorrow. His car is completely out of gas. His bike has a flat tire.
> → *He could take the bus to work.*
> → *He could get a friend to take him to a gas station to get gas.*
> → *He could try to fix his bike.*
> → *He could get up very early and walk to work.*
>   *Etc.*

1. Lisa walked to school today. Now she wants to go home. It's raining hard. She doesn't have an umbrella, and she's wearing sandals.
2. Joe and Joan want to get some exercise. They were planning to play tennis this morning, but it snowed last night, and the tennis court is full of snow.
3. Roberto just bought a new TV. He has it at home now. The remote control is complicated. It has a lot of buttons. He doesn't understand how to use all of them.
4. Albert is traveling around the world. He is 22 years old. Today he is alone in Paris. He needs to eat, and he needs to find a place to stay overnight. But while he was asleep on the train last night, someone stole his wallet. He has no money and no credit cards.

EXERCISE 17 ▸ Listening. (Charts 7-3 and 7-4)

Listen to the conversation between a husband and wife. Listen again and complete the sentences with the words you hear.

In a Home Office

A: Look at this cord. Do you know what it's for?

B: I don't know. We have so many cables and cords around here with all our electronic equipment.

It _____ for our old printer.

1

A: No, that isn't a printer cord.

B: It _____ for one of the kids' toys.

2

A: Yeah, I _____. But they don't have

3
many electronic toys.

B: I have an idea. It _____ for an old

4
cell phone. You know — the one I had before this one.

A: I bet that's it. We _____ probably throw this out.

5

B: Well, let's be sure before we do that.

EXERCISE 18 ▶ Looking at grammar. (Charts 7-2 → 7-4)
Choose the verb that has the same meaning as the phrase in **bold**. More than one answer may be correct.

1. Thomas **is able to** memorize long numbers. He   can / could   remember a lot.

2. **It's possible** the weather will be nice tomorrow. It   might / may   be sunny.

3. You **have** my **permission** to stay out late. You   can / may   stay out until 1:00 A.M.

4. **Were you able to** read the doctor's note?   Can / Could   you read her handwriting?

5. Julia isn't here. **It's possible** she's at home. She   was able to / could   still be asleep.

6. I **wasn't able to** go to the dance. I hurt my foot, and I   couldn't / may not   dance.

7. **Are you able to** find a computer virus and remove it?   May / Can   you get rid of a computer virus?

EXERCISE 19 ▶ Warm-up. (Chart 7-5)
Check (✓) all the grammatically correct sentences.

At the Airport

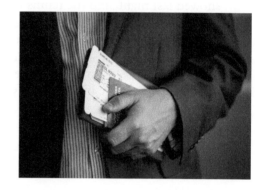

1. _____ May I see your ID and boarding pass?

2. _____ Can I see your ID and boarding pass?

3. _____ Could I see your ID and boarding pass?

4. _____ May you show me your ID and boarding pass?

7-5 Polite Requests with *I: May, Could, Can*

Polite Request	Possible Answers	
(a) *May I* please borrow your pen? (b) *Could I* please borrow your pen? (c) *Can I* please borrow your pen?	Yes. Yes. Of course. Yes. Certainly. Of course. Certainly. Sure. (*informal*) OK. (*informal*) Uh-huh. (*meaning "yes"*) I'm sorry, but I need to use it myself.	People use *may*, *could*, and *can* to make polite requests with *I*.* The questions ask for someone's permission or agreement. Examples (a), (b), and (c) have basically the same meaning. *Can I* is less formal than *may I* and *could I*. NOTE: *May* is not used with *you* in polite requests.
(d) *Can I* borrow your pen, please? (e) *Can I* borrow your pen?		*Please* can come at the end of the question, as in (d). *Please* can be omitted from the question, as in (e).

*In a polite question, *could* is NOT the past form of *can*.

EXERCISE 20 ▸ Grammar and speaking. (Chart 7-5)
Complete the phone conversations. Use *May I*, *Could I*, or *Can I* + a verb in the box.
NOTE: The caller is always Speaker B. Practice your conversations with a partner.

ask	help	leave	reschedule	speak/talk

Hello?

1. A: Hello?

   B: Hello. Is Ahmed there?

   A: Yes, he is.

   B: _____ to him?

   A: Just a minute. I'll get him.

2. A: Hello? Mr. Black's office.

   B: _____ to Mr. Black?

   A: _____ who is calling?

   B: Susan Abbott.

   A: Just a moment, Ms. Abbott. I'll transfer you.

3. A: Hello?

   B: Hi. This is Bob. _____ to Pedro?

   A: Sure. Hold on.

4. A: Good afternoon. Dr. Wu's office. _____ you?

   B: Yes. I have an appointment that I need to change.

   A: Just a minute, please. I'll transfer you to our appointment desk.

5. A: Hello?

   B: Hi Emily. It's Nina. I'm still at work and can't leave. _____
   our appointment.

   A: Sure. Let me get my calendar.

6. A: Hello?

   B: Hello. _____ to Maria?

   A: She's not here right now.

   B: Oh. _____ a message?

   A: Sure. Just let me get a pen.

EXERCISE 21 ▸ Let's talk: pairwork. (Chart 7-5)

Work with a partner. Ask and answer polite questions. Begin with *May I*, *Could I*, or *Can I*. Make conversations you can perform for the class.

Polite Requests

Example: (A), you want to see (B)'s grammar book for a minute.
PARTNER A: May/Could/Can I (please) see your grammar book for a minute?
PARTNER B: Of course. / Sure. / Etc.
PARTNER A: Thank you. / Thanks. I forgot to bring mine to class today.

1. (A), you want to see (B)'s dictionary for a minute.
2. (B), you are on the phone with (A). Someone knocks on your door. You want to call (A) back.
3. (A), you are at a restaurant. (B) is your server. You have finished your meal. You want the check.
4. (B), you run into (A) on the street. (A) is carrying some heavy packages. What are you going to say to him/her?
5. (A), you are speaking to (B), who is one of your teachers. You aren't feeling well and want to leave class early today.
6. (B), you are in a store with your good friend (A). You go to pay for your groceries, but you left your wallet at home.
7. (A), you are paying for an item in a store. (B) is the cashier. You want to pay with a check, but you don't know if the store takes checks.

EXERCISE 22 ▸ Warm-up. (Chart 7-6)

Check (✓) all the correct requests.

There are a lot of dishes tonight.

1. _____ Will you help me with the dishes?
2. _____ Would you load the dishwasher?
3. _____ May you load the dishwasher?
4. _____ Can you unload the dishwasher?
5. _____ Could you unload the dishwasher?

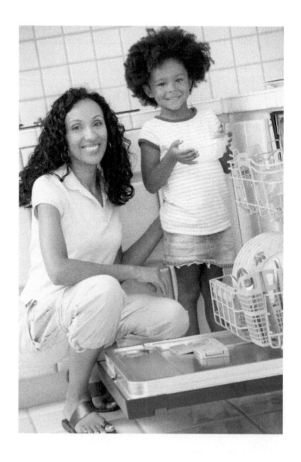

7-6 Polite Requests with *You: Would, Could, Will, Can*

Polite Requests	Possible Answers	
(a) *Would you* please open the door? (b) *Could you* please open the door? (c) *Will you* please open the door? (d) *Can you* please open the door?	Yes. Yes. Of course. Certainly. I'd be happy to. Of course. I'd be glad to. Sure. (*informal*) OK. (*informal*) Uh-huh. (*meaning* "yes") I'm sorry. I'd like to help, but my hands are full.	People use *would*, *could*, *will* and *can* with *you* to make polite requests. The questions ask for someone's help or cooperation. Examples (a), (b), (c), and (d) have basically the same meaning. *Would* and *could* sound a little more formal than *will* and *can*. For some speakers, *would* and *could* sound more polite, but tone of voice and the use of *please* can also determine politeness.
		NOTE: *May* is NOT used when *you* is the subject of a polite request. *INCORRECT:* *May you please open the door?*

EXERCISE 23 ▶ Looking at grammar. (Chart 7-6)
Make two different questions for each situation. Use *you*.

1. You're in a room and it's getting very hot.

   Formal: _____Would you please open the window?_____

   Informal: _____Can you turn on the air conditioner?_____

2. You're trying to watch TV, but your friends are talking too loud, and you can't hear it.

   Formal: _____

   Informal: _____

3. You're in a restaurant. You are about to pay and notice the bill is more than it should be. The server has made a mistake.

   Formal: _____

   Informal: _____

4. You are in an apartment building and running toward an elevator. There is a woman in it, and the door is beginning to close. You want her to hold it open for you.

   Formal: _____

   Informal: _____

EXERCISE 24 ▶ Let's talk: pairwork. (Charts 7-5 and 7-6)
Work with a partner. Make a conversation for one (or more) of the situations. Perform your conversation for the rest of the class.

Example: You're in a restaurant. You want the server to refill your coffee cup. You catch the server's eye and raise your hand slightly. He approaches your table and says: "Yes? What can I do for you?"

PARTNER A: Yes? What can I do for you?
PARTNER B: Could I please have some more coffee?
PARTNER A: Of course. Right away. Could I get you anything else?
PARTNER B: No thanks. Oh, on second thought, yes. Would you bring some cream too?
PARTNER A: Certainly.
PARTNER B: Thanks.

1. You've been waiting in a long line at a busy bakery. Finally, it's your turn. The clerk turns toward you and says: "Next!"

2. You are at work. You feel sick and you have a slight fever. You really want to go home. You see your boss, Mr. Jenkins, walking by your desk. You say: "Mr. Jenkins, could I speak with you for a minute?"

3. The person next to you on the plane has a bag on the floor that is in your space. You would like him to move it. You say: "Excuse me."

EXERCISE 25 ▶ Looking at grammar. (Charts 7-5 and 7-6)
Choose the correct verbs. In some cases, both answers may be correct.

At a Government Office

1. _____ your name please?
   a. May I have   b. May you give me

2. _____ your driver's license or passport?
   a. Can I see   b. Could you show me

3. _____ take your driver's license out of your wallet?
   a. Will you   b. Can you

4. _____ write down your address?
   a. May you   b. Could you

5. _____ please sign your name on the line?
   a. Will you   b. Would you

6. _____ also write the date?
   a. Can you   b. May you

7. _____ tell me the best way to reach you?
   a. May you   b. Would you

EXERCISE 26 ▸ Warm-up. (Chart 7-7)
Your friend Paula has a terrible headache. What advice would you give her?
Check (✓) the sentences you agree with.

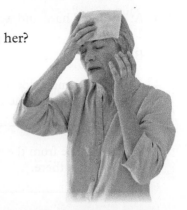

1. _____ You should lie down.

2. _____ You should take some medicine.

3. _____ You ought to call the doctor.

4. _____ You should go to the emergency room.

5. _____ You ought to put an ice-pack on your forehead.

7-7	Expressing Advice: *Should* and *Ought To*

(a) My clothes are dirty. I { *should* / *ought to* } wash them.	*Should* and *ought to* have the same meaning: "This is a good idea. This is good advice."
	
	 FORMS:
	    should + simple form of a verb (no *to*)
	    ought + *to* + simple form of a verb

(b) INCORRECT: *I should to wash them.* (c) INCORRECT: *I ought washing them.*	
(d) You need your sleep. You *should not* (*shouldn't*) stay up late.	NEGATIVE: *should* + *not* = *shouldn't* (*Ought to* is usually not used in the negative.)
(e) A: I'm going to be late for the bus. What *should I do*? B: Run!	QUESTION: *should* + *subject* + *main verb* (*Ought to* is usually not used in questions.)
(f) A: I'm tired today. B: You *should/ought to* go home and take a nap.	The use of *maybe* with *should* and *ought to* "softens" advice. COMPARE: In (f): Speaker B is giving definite advice. He is stating clearly that he believes going home for a nap is a good idea and is the solution to Speaker A's problem.
(g) A: I'm tired today. B: *Maybe* you *should/ought to* go home and take a nap.	In (g): Speaker B is making a suggestion: going home for a nap is one possible way to solve Speaker A's problem.

EXERCISE 27 ▸ Let's talk: pairwork. (Chart 7-7)
Complete the conversations with ***should*** or ***ought to***.

Giving Advice

1. A: My computer has started to make a buzzing noise. I just bought it last month.

   B: You _____ .

2. A: For the past week, I've woken up every morning with a stiff neck. I can't figure out why. I'm not sleeping differently. My mattress and pillow are the same.

   B: You _____ .

3. A: I worked hard and wrote a really good paper for history. My teacher doesn't think I wrote it, but I did.

   B: You _____ .

4. A: My roommate doesn't clean up. The kitchen sink is full of his dirty dishes. His clothes are all over the apartment. I've talked to him many times about this.

   B: You _____ .

5. A: I got home from the store and found a shirt in my bag. I didn't buy it. My four-year old son had put it there.

   B: You _____ .

6. A: My daughter's friend takes really long showers when she stays with us. Sometimes she uses all the hot water.

   B: You _____ .

EXERCISE 28 ▶ Let's talk: pairwork. (Chart 7-7)

Work with a partner. Partner A states the problem. Partner B gives advice using **should** or **ought to**. Include **maybe** to soften the advice if you wish. Take turns. Look at your partner before you speak.

Example: I'm sleepy.
PARTNER A: I'm sleepy.
PARTNER B: (Maybe) You should drink/ought to drink some coffee.

PARTNER A	PARTNER B
1. I can't fall asleep at night.	5. I'm starving.★
2. I have a sore throat.	6. I have the hiccups.
3. I dropped my sister's phone and cracked the screen.	7. Someone stole my lunch from the refrigerator in the staff lounge at work.
4. I sat on my friend's sunglasses. Now the frames are bent.	8. I bought some shoes that don't fit. Now my feet hurt.
	Change roles.

EXERCISE 29 ▶ Warm-up. (Chart 7-8)

Marco lost his passport. Here are some suggestions. Check (✓) the sentences you agree with. Which sentences seem more serious or urgent?

1. _____ He had better go to the embassy.

2. _____ He should wait and see if someone returns it.

3. _____ He had better report it to the police.

4. _____ He should ask a friend to help him look for it.

★*starving* (informal English) = very, very hungry

7-8 Expressing Advice: *Had Better*

(a) My clothes are dirty. I $\left\{\begin{array}{l}\textit{should}\\\textit{ought to}\\\textit{had better}\end{array}\right\}$ *wash* them.	**Had better** has the same basic meaning as *should* and *ought to*: "This is a good idea. This is good advice."
(b) You're driving too fast! You**'d better** *slow* down.	**Had better** has more of a sense of urgency than *should* or *ought to*. It often implies a warning about possible bad consequences. In (b): If you don't slow down, there could be a bad result. You could get a speeding ticket or have an accident.
(c) You**'d better not** *eat* that meat. It looks spoiled.	NEGATIVE: **had better not**
(d) I**'d better** *send* my boss an email right away.	In conversation, **had** is usually contracted: **'d**.

EXERCISE 30 ▸ Grammar and speaking. (Chart 7-8)

Give advice using ***had better***. Then mention some bad consequences if the person doesn't follow the advice. Work in pairs, in small groups, or as a class.

1. I haven't paid my electric bill.
   → *You'd better pay it by tomorrow. If you don't pay it, the electric company will turn off the power.*

2. Joe oversleeps a lot. This week he has been late to work three times. His boss is very unhappy about that.

3. I don't feel good right now. I think I'm coming down with something.★

4. I can't remember if I locked the front door when I left for work.

5. I can't find my credit card, and I've looked everywhere.

6. My ankle really hurts. I think I've sprained it.

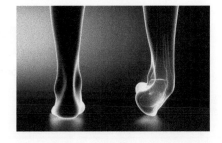

EXERCISE 31 ▸ Let's talk. (Charts 7-7 and 7-8)

Work in small groups. Give advice using ***should***, ***ought to***, and ***had better***. The leader states the problem, and others in the group offer suggestions. Select a different leader for each item on page 210.

Example:

LEADER: I study, but I don't understand my physics class. It's the middle of the term, and I'm failing the course. I need a science course in order to graduate. What should I do?★★

STUDENT A: You**'d better** get a tutor right away.

STUDENT B: You **should** make an appointment with your teacher and see if you can get some extra help.

STUDENT C: Maybe you **ought to** drop your physics course and take a different science course next term.

★The idiom *come down with something* = get sick.

★★*Should* (NOT *ought to* or *had better*) is usually used in a question that asks for advice. The answer, however, can contain *should, ought to,* or *had better.* For example:

A: *My houseplants always die. What **should** I do?*

B: *You**'d better** get a book on plants. You **should** try to find out why they die. Maybe you **ought to** look on the internet and see if you can find some information.*

1. I forgot my dad's birthday yesterday. I feel terrible about it. What should I do?

2. I just discovered that I made dinner plans for tonight with two different people. I'm supposed to meet my parents at one restaurant at 7:00, and I'm supposed to meet my boss at a different restaurant across town at 8:00. What should I do?

3. Samira accidentally left the grocery store with an item she didn't pay for. It was under her purse in the shopping cart. What should Samira do?

4. I borrowed Karen's favorite book of poetry. It was special to her. A note on the inside cover said "To Karen." The author's signature was under it. Now I can't find the book. I think I lost it. What should I do?

EXERCISE 32 ▶ Warm-up. (Chart 7-9)

Which of these statements about writing a résumé are true in your country? Check (✓) them. Which sentence is more common in writing? Which sentences are more common in speaking?

Writing a Résumé

1. _____ You must list all your previous employers.

2. _____ You have to provide references.

3. _____ You have got to include personal information, for example, whether you are married or not.

7-9	Expressing Necessity: *Have To, Have Got To, Must*

(a) I have a very important test tomorrow. I { *have to* / *have got to* / *must* } *study* tonight.	*Have to*, *have got to*, and *must* have basically the same meaning. They express the idea that something is necessary.
(b) I'd like to go with you to the movie this evening, but I can't. I *have to go* to a meeting. (c) Bye now! I*'ve got to go*. My wife's waiting for me. I'll call you later. (d) All passengers *must present* their passports at customs upon arrival. (e) Tommy, you *must hold* onto the railing when you go down the stairs.	*Have to* is used much more frequently in everyday speech and writing than *must*. *Have got to* is typically used in informal conversation, as in (c). *Must* is typically found in written instructions or rules, as in (d). Adults also use it when talking to younger children, as in (e). It sounds very strong.
(f) *Do* we *have to bring* pencils to the test? (g) Why *did* he *have to leave* so early?	QUESTIONS: *Have to* is usually used in questions, not *must* or *have got to*. Forms of *do* are used with *have to* in questions.
(h) I *had to study* last night.	The PAST form of *have to*, *have got to*, and *must* (meaning necessity) is *had to*. NOTE: *Must* is NOT used for the past tense.
(i) I *have to* ("hafta") *go* downtown today. (j) Rita *has to* ("hasta") *go* to the bank. (k) I*'ve got to* ("gotta") *study* tonight.	NOTE: *Have to*, *has to*, and *have got to* are commonly reduced, as in (i) through (k).

EXERCISE 33 ▶ Grammar and speaking. (Charts 7-7 and 7-9)
Choose the correct meaning for each statement. Which ones do you agree with?

Rules or Advice?

1.	Teenagers have to be respectful to their parents.	necessity	advice
2.	The elderly should live with their children.	necessity	advice
3.	Babies ought to sleep with their mothers.	necessity	advice
4.	Kids have got to obey their parents.	necessity	advice
5.	Families should have dinner together every night.	necessity	advice
6.	Parents must love their children.	necessity	advice

EXERCISE 34 ▶ Let's talk. (Charts 7-7 and 7-9)
Answer the questions. Work in pairs, in small groups, or as a class.

1. What are some things you have to do today? Tomorrow? Every day?
2. What is something you had to do yesterday?
3. What is something you've got to do soon?
4. What is something you've got to do after class today or later tonight?
5. What is something a driver must do, according to the law?
6. What is something a safe driver should or shouldn't do?
7. What are some things a person should or shouldn't do to stay healthy?
8. What are some things a person must do to stay alive?

EXERCISE 35 ▶ Grammar and speaking. (Charts 7-7 and 7-9)
Check (✓) the statement in each pair that you agree with. Discuss your answers with another student or in small groups.

At a Restaurant

1. _____ Diners must leave a tip.

   _____ Diners should leave a tip.

2. _____ Servers must wash their hands.

   _____ Servers ought to wash their hands.

3. _____ People have got to put their phones away in the restaurant.

   _____ People should put their phones away in the restaurant.

4. _____ The restaurant manager should greet customers when they enter the restaurant.

   _____ The restaurant manager has to greet customers when they enter the restaurant.

5. _____ The servers must wear uniforms.

   _____ The servers should wear their own clothes.

EXERCISE 36 ▶ Looking at grammar. (Charts 7-2 → 7-4, 7-7, and 7-9)

Part I. Choose the correct completions for the sentences. Sometimes both choices may be correct.

Many English names have two forms: a formal or legal name and an informal one.

For example, you   should / may   know a person as Andy, but his legal name is Andrew.
                      ¹
Or, for a woman, Kathy   could / may   have the formal name Katherine or Kathleen.
                            ²
Why is this important? Imagine you   have to / maybe   look up a phone number, either in a
                                         ³
phone book or on the internet. People   might / can   use their formal name for registration, and
                                           ⁴
this   could / may   show up on the internet or elsewhere.
         ⁵
   Look at these names: Nick, Lilly.   Can you / Are you able to   give the formal names?
                                          ⁶

Part II. Work with a partner. Write a formal name for each of the following.

1. Bob, Bobby → _____   5. Debbie → _____

2. Danny → _____   6. Sue → _____

3. Jon, Jonny → _____   7. Alex → _____

4. Bill, Billy → _____   8. Terry → _____

EXERCISE 37 ▶ Listening. (Chart 7-9)
Complete the sentences with the words you hear.

EMPLOYMENT APPLICATION

Applications are considered for all positions without regard to race, color, religion, sex, national origin, age, marital or veteran status, or in the presence of a non-related medical condition or handicap.

Donna	N/A	Frost	May 4, 2019
First Name	Middle Initial	Last Name	Date

1443 Maple Ridge Heights	052-555-5454
Address	Phone #

Happyville	PA	04321	123-000-7890
City	State	Zip Code	Social Security #

Do you know these words?
- employment   - previous
- applicable   - employer
- legal   - apply
- nickname

Filling out a Job Application

1. The application _____ be complete. You shouldn't skip any parts. If a section doesn't fit your situation, you can write N/A (not applicable).

2. If you fill out the form by hand, your writing _____ be easy to read.

3. _____ use your full legal name, not your nickname.

4. _____ list the names and places of your previous employers.

5. _____ list your education, beginning with either high school or college.

6. All spelling _____ be correct.

7. A: _____ write the same thing twice, like a phone number?

   B: No, you can just write "same as above."

8. A: _____ apply in person?

   B: No, for a lot of companies, you can do it online.

EXERCISE 38 ▸ Reading and speaking. (Charts 7-7 → 7-9)
Part I. Read the passage.

A Family Problem

Mr. and Mrs. Hill don't know what to do about their 15-year-old son, Mark. He's very intelligent but has no interest in learning. His grades are getting worse, and he won't do any homework. Sometimes he skips school and spends the day at the mall.

His older sister Kathy is a good student, and she never causes any problems at home. Kathy hasn't missed a day of school all year. Mark's parents keep asking him why he can't be more like Kathy. Mark is jealous of Kathy and picks fights* with her.

All Mark likes to do is stay in his bedroom and listen to loud music or play video games. He often refuses to eat meals with his family. He argues with his parents, his room is a mess, and he won't** help around the house.

Part II. This family needs advice. Work with a partner. What should they do? What shouldn't they do? Make a list, and compare your suggestions with the advice of other classmates.

Use each of these words at least once in the advice you give.

should	have got to/has got to	ought to	must
shouldn't	had better	have to/has to	

EXERCISE 39 ▸ Warm-up. (Chart 7-10)
Which sentence (a. or b.) completes the idea of the given sentence?

We have lots of time.
   a. You must not hurry!
   b. You don't have to hurry!

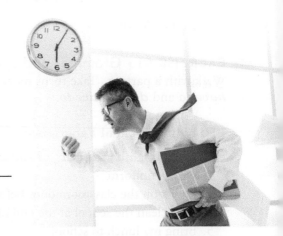

---

*pick a fight = start a fight

**won't is used here to express refusal: *He refuses to help around the house.*

7-10 Expressing Lack of Necessity: *Do Not Have To;* Expressing Prohibition: *Must Not*

(a) I finished all of my homework this afternoon. I *don't have to study* tonight. (b) Tomorrow is a holiday. Mary *doesn't have to go* to class. (c) I *didn't have to work* last week. I had several days off.	***Don't / doesn't / didn't have to*** express the idea that something is *not necessary*.
(d) Bus passengers *must not talk* to the driver. (e) Tommy, you *must not/mustn't* play* with matches! (f) *Do not/Don't* talk to the driver. (g) *Do not/Don't* play with matches.	***Must not*** expresses *prohibition* (DO NOT DO THIS!). ***Must not*** is not common; it is generally used for rules or with children. Speakers more often express prohibition with imperatives**, as in (f) and (g).

  *The first "t" is not pronounced.
**See also Chart 7-13.

EXERCISE 40 ▶ Looking at grammar. (Chart 7-10)
Complete the sentences with ***don't have to, doesn't have to,*** or ***must not***.

1. You _____*must not*_____ drive when you are tired. It's dangerous.

2. I live only a few blocks from my office. I _____*don't have to*_____ drive to work.

3. Liz finally got a car, so now she drives to work. She _____ take the bus.

4. Mr. Murphy is very wealthy. He _____ work for a living.

5. You _____ tell Daddy about the birthday party. We want it to be a surprise.

6. A: Did Professor Acosta give an assignment?

   B: Yes, she assigned Chapters 4 and 6, but we _____ read Chapter 5.

7. A: Listen carefully, Kristen. If a stranger offers you a ride, you _____ get in the car. Never get in a car with a stranger. Do you understand?

   B: Yes, Mom.

EXERCISE 41 ▶ Grammar and speaking. (Charts 7-9 and 7-10)
Work with a partner. Take turns making true sentences about your time in elementary school using ***have to*** and ***didn't have to***.

Elementary School Experiences

1. study English grammar → *I had to / didn't have to study English grammar.*
2. wear a uniform
3. knock on the classroom door before I entered
4. help clean the school at the end of the day
5. bring my lunch to school

6. learn keyboarding skills for the computer
7. take a lot of tests
8. use online textbooks
9. sing by myself in front of other students
10. do a lot of homework every night

EXERCISE 42 ▸ Warm-up. (Chart 7-11)
Read the situation and the conclusions that follow. Which conclusion(s) seem(s) logical to you?
Explain your answers, if necessary.

SITUATION: Mr. Ellis is a high school gym teacher. He usually wears gym clothes to work.
Today he is wearing a suit and tie.

1. He must have an important meeting.
2. He must be rich.
3. He must need new clothes.

4. He must want to make a good impression on someone.
5. His gym clothes must not be clean.

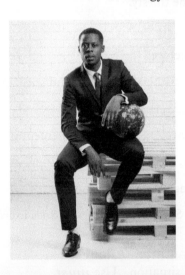

7-11 Making Logical Conclusions: *Must*	
(a) A: Nancy is yawning. B: She *must be* sleepy.	In (a): Speaker B is making a logical guess. He bases his guess on the information that Nancy is yawning. His logical conclusion, his "best guess," is that Nancy is sleepy. He uses ***must*** to express his logical conclusion.
(b) LOGICAL CONCLUSION: Lea doesn't eat meat. She *must be* *vegetarian*. (c) NECESSITY: If you want to get into the movie theater, you *must buy* a ticket.	COMPARE: ***Must*** can express • a logical conclusion, as in (b). • necessity, as in (c).
(d) NEGATIVE LOGICAL CONCLUSION: Eric ate everything on his plate except the pickle. He *must not like* pickles. (e) PROHIBITION: There are sharks near the hotel beach. You *must not go* swimming there.	COMPARE: ***Must not*** can express • a negative logical conclusion, as in (d). • prohibition, as in (e).

EXERCISE 43 ▶ Looking at grammar. (Chart 7-11)
Complete the conversations with *must* or *must not*.

My Best Guess

1. A: Did you offer our guests something to eat?

   B: Yes, but they didn't want anything. They ___*must not*___ be hungry yet.

2. A: You haven't eaten since breakfast? That was hours ago. You ___*must*___ be hungry.

   B: I am.

3. A: Gregory has already had four glasses of water, and now he's having another.

   B: He _____ be really thirsty.

4. A: I offered Holly something to drink, but she doesn't want anything.

   B: She _____ be thirsty.

5. A: The dog won't eat.

   B: He _____ feel well.

6. A: Brian has watery eyes and has been coughing and sneezing.

   B: Poor guy. He _____ have a cold.

7. A: Erica's really smart. She always gets above 95 percent on her math tests.

   B: I'm sure she's pretty bright, but she _____ also study a lot.

8. A: Listen. Someone is jumping on the floor above us.

   B: It _____ be Sam. Sometimes he does exercises in his apartment.

EXERCISE 44 ▶ Looking at grammar. (Chart 7-11)
Make a logical conclusion for each situation. Use *must*.

1. Alima is crying. → *She must be unhappy.*
2. Mrs. Chu has a big smile on her face.
3. Samantha is shivering.
4. Olga watches ten movies a week.
5. James is sweating.
6. Toshi can lift one end of a compact car by himself.

EXERCISE 45 ▶ Let's talk. (Chart 7-11)
Make logical conclusions with *must* or *must not*. Use the suggested phrases and/or your own words.

1. I am at Cyril's apartment door. I've knocked on the door and have rung the doorbell several times. Nobody has answered the door. (*be at home? be out somewhere?*)
   → *Cyril must not be at home. He must be out somewhere.*

2. Jennifer reads all the time. She sits in a quiet corner and reads even when people come to visit her. (*love books? like books better than people? like to talk to people?*)

3. Lara has a full academic schedule, plays on the volleyball team, takes piano lessons, and has a part-time job at an ice-cream store. (*be busy all the time? have a lot of spare time? be a hard worker?*)

4. Simon gets on the internet every day as soon as he gets home from work. He stays at his computer until he goes to bed. (*be a computer addict? have a happy home life? have a lot of friends?*)

EXERCISE 46 ▸ Looking at grammar. (Charts 7-9 and 7-11)
Complete the sentences with *must, have to,* or *had to* and the correct form of the verbs in parentheses.

At Work

A: Your eyes are red. You (*be*) _____ really tired.
₁

B: Yeah, I (*stay*) _____ up all night working on a project.
₂

A: Did you finish?

B: No, I (*work*) _____ on it later today, but I have a million other things to do.
₃

A: You (*be*) _____ really busy.
₄

B: I am!

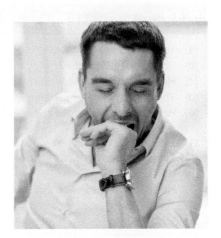

EXERCISE 47 ▸ Looking at grammar. (Charts 7-7 → 7-11)
Choose the verb that has the same meaning as the phrase in **bold**. More than one answer may be correct.

Buying a Car

1. You really **don't have a choice**. You   have to / should   test-drive the car before you buy it.

2. **It's a good idea** to get information about cars on the internet before you go to the dealer. You   should / must   find out about things like reliability ratings and paying a fair price.

3. You **don't need to** buy a car today. You   don't have to / must not   make your decision right now. You can take some time and shop around.

4. You **need to** find out the insurance costs. You   have got to / have to   call your insurance company first. Some cars are very expensive to insure.

5. **It's a bad idea** to pay full price for a car. You   shouldn't / couldn't   pay the sticker price.

6. **That's my best guess**. The price is low. The dealer   must / had better   want to sell it quickly.

7. **That's a good idea**. You   ought to / should   find out the invoice price (the price the dealer pays for the car) before you make an offer.

EXERCISE 48 ▸ Warm-up. (Chart 7-12)

Complete the questions with the correct words in the box. Two words don't fit any questions.

can't	couldn't	do	does	will	wouldn't

1. You can work this weekend, _____ you?

2. He won't be late, _____ he?

3. We'd like you to stay, _____ we?

4. They don't have to leave, _____ they?

7-12 Tag Questions with Modal Auxiliaries

(a) You *can* come, ***can't you***? (b) She *won't* tell, ***will she***? (c) He *should* help, ***shouldn't he***? (d) They *couldn't* do it, ***could they***? (e) We *would like* to help, ***wouldn't we***?	Tag questions are common with these modal auxiliaries: ***can, will, should, could,*** and ***would***.*
(f) They *have to* leave, ***don't they***? (g) They *don't have to* leave, ***do they***? (h) He *has to* leave, ***doesn't he***? (i) He *doesn't have to* leave, ***does he***? (j) You *had to* leave, ***didn't you***? (k) You *didn't have to* leave, ***did you***?	Tag questions are also common with ***have to, has to,*** and ***had to***. Notice that forms of ***do*** are used for the tag in (f) through (k).

*See Chart 5-13, p. 149, for information on how to use tag questions.

EXERCISE 49 ▸ Looking at grammar. (Chart 7-12)

Complete the tag questions.

1. You can answer these questions, _____ you?

2. Melinda won't tell anyone our secret, _____ she?

3. Alice would like to come with us, _____ she?

4. I don't have to do more chores, _____ I?

5. Steven shouldn't come to the meeting, _____ he?

6. Flies can fly upside down, _____ they?

7. You would rather have your own apartment, _____ you?

8. Jill has to renew her driver's license, _____ she?

9. If you want to catch your bus, you should leave now, _____ you?

10. Ms. Baxter will be here tomorrow, _____ she?

11. You couldn't hear me, _____ you?

12. We had to work hard in our chemistry class, _____ we?

EXERCISE 50 ▶ Warm-up. (Chart 7-13)

Read each group of sentences. Decide who the speaker is and a possible situation for each group.

GROUP A

1. Show me your driver's license.
2. Take it out of your wallet, please.
3. Give me your registration and proof of insurance.
4. Step out of the car.

GROUP B

1. Open your mouth.
2. Stick out your tongue.
3. Say "ahhh."
4. Let me take a closer look.
5. Don't bite me!

7-13 Imperative Sentences: Giving Instructions

COMMAND: (a) Captain: *Open* the door! Soldier: Yes, sir! REQUEST: (b) Teacher: *Open* the door, please. Student: Sure. DIRECTIONS: (c) Barbara: Could you tell me how to get to the post office? Stranger: Sure. *Walk* two blocks down this street. *Turn* left *and walk* three more blocks. It's on the right-hand side of the street.	Imperative sentences are used to give commands, make polite requests, and give directions. The difference between a command and a request lies in the speaker's tone of voice and the use of **please**. **Please** can come at the beginning or end of a request: *Open the door, please.* *Please open the door.* INCORRECT: *You open the door please.*
(d) *Close* the window. (e) Please *sit* down. (f) *Be* quiet! (g) *Don't walk* on the grass. (h) Please *don't wait* for me. (i) *Don't be* late.	The simple form of a verb is used in imperative sentences. In (d): The understood subject of the sentence is **you** (meaning the person the speaker is talking to): *Close the window = You close the window.* NEGATIVE FORM: **Don't** + the simple form of a verb

EXERCISE 51 ▶ Let's talk. (Chart 7-13)

Part I. Work with a partner or in small groups. Read the steps for cooking rice. Put them in a logical order (1–8).

Cooking Rice

a. _____ Measure the rice.

b. _____ Cook for 20 minutes.

c. _____ Pour water into a pan.

d. _____ Bring the water to a boil.

e. _____ Put the rice in the pan.

f. _____ Set the timer.

g. _____ Turn off the heat.

h. _____ Take the pan off the stove.

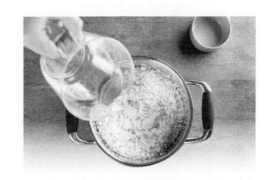

Part II. Write instructions for cooking something simple. Share your recipe with the class.

EXERCISE 52 ▶ Listening. (Chart 7-13)

Part I. Listen to the steps in this number puzzle, and write the verbs you hear.

Do you know these words?
- double
- add
- multiply
- subtract

Puzzle steps:

1. _____ down the number of the month you were born. For example,

_____ the number 2 if you were born in February.

_____ 3 if you were born in March, etc.

2. _____ the number.

3. _____ 5 to it.

4. _____ it by 50.

5. _____ your age.

6. _____ 250.

Part II. Now follow the steps in Part I to complete the puzzle. In the final number, the last two digits on the right will be your age, and the one or two digits on the left will be the month you were born.

EXERCISE 53 ▶ Warm-up. (Chart 7-14)
Check (✓) the sentences that are suggestions.

1. _____ Why do bears hibernate?

2. _____ I have a day off. Why don't we take the kids to the zoo?

3. _____ Let's go see the bears at the zoo.

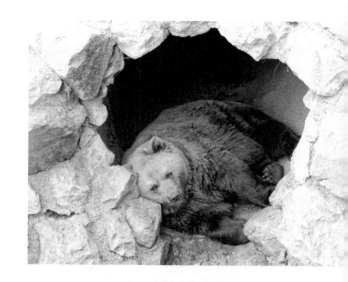

7-14 Making Suggestions: *Let's* and *Why Don't*

(a)   — It's hot today. *Let's go to the beach*.
      — OK. Good idea.
 	
(b)   — It's hot today. *Why don't we go to the beach*?
      — OK. Good idea.
	Let's and **Why don't we** are used to make suggestions about activities for you and another person or other people to do.
	Examples (a) and (b) have the same meaning.
	Let's = *let us*

(c)   — I'm tired.
      — *Why don't you take a nap*?
      — That's a good idea. I think I will.
	In (c): **Why don't you** is used to make a friendly suggestion or to give friendly advice.

EXERCISE 54 ▶ Looking at grammar. (Chart 7-14)
Choose the sentences that can be suggestions.

1. a. Why don't you wear something different today?
   b. Why do you wear red on Mondays?

2. a. Why did you get to work late?
   b. Why didn't you get to work on time?
   c. Why don't we get to work early?

3. a. Why do you only check email at night?
   b. Why don't you check your email now?

EXERCISE 55 ▶ Let's talk. (Chart 7-14)
Make suggestions beginning with **Let's** and **Why don't we**.

Dinner Plans

1. Where should we go for dinner tonight?
2. Who should we ask to join us for dinner tonight?
3. What time should we meet at the restaurant?
4. Where should we go afterwards?

EXERCISE 56 ▶ Let's talk. (Chart 7-14)
Work in small groups. One person states the problem, and then others in the group offer suggestions beginning with **Why don't you**.

Help!

1. I'm freezing.
2. I'm feeling dizzy.
3. I'm so bored. I want to do something fun this weekend. Any ideas?
4. I've lost my last cell phone charger. I had three, and now I have none.
5. I haven't done my assignment for Professor Lopez. It will take me a couple of hours, and class starts in an hour. What am I going to do?

6. I've lost the key to my apartment, so I can't get in. My roommate is at the library. What am I going to do?

7. My friend and I had an argument, and now we aren't talking to each other. I've had some time to think about it, and I'm sorry for what I said. I miss her friendship. What should I do?

EXERCISE 57 ▸ Warm-up. (Chart 7-15)
Check (✓) the statements that are true for you.

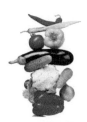

1. _____ I prefer vegetables to fruit.

2. _____ I like raw vegetables better than cooked.

3. _____ I would rather eat vegetables than meat.

7-15 Stating Preferences: *Prefer, Like ... Better, Would Rather*

(a) I *prefer* apples *to* oranges. (b) I *prefer* watching TV *to* studying.	**prefer** + *noun* + **to** + *noun* **prefer** + **-ing** *verb* + **to** + **-ing** *verb*
(c) I *like* apples *better than* oranges. (d) I *like* watching TV *better than* studying.	**like** + *noun* + **better than** + *noun* **like** + **-ing** *verb* + **better than** + **-ing** *verb*
(e) Ann *would rather have* an apple than an orange. (f) INCORRECT: *Ann would rather has an apple.* (g) I'd rather visit a big city *than live* there. (h) INCORRECT: *I'd rather visit a big city than to live there.* INCORRECT: *I'd rather visit a big city than living there.*	**Would rather** is followed immediately by the simple form of a verb (e.g., *have, visit, live*), as in (e). Verbs following **than** are also in the simple form, as in (g).
(i) *I'd / You'd / She'd / He'd / We'd / They'd* rather have an apple.	Contraction of **would** = **'d**
(j) *Would you rather* have an apple *or* an orange?	In (j): In a polite question, **would rather** can be followed by **or** to offer someone a choice.

EXERCISE 58 ▸ Looking at grammar. (Chart 7-15)
Complete the sentences with **than** or **to**.

1. When I'm hot and thirsty, I prefer cold drinks ___to___ hot drinks.

2. When I'm hot and thirsty, I like cold drinks better ___than___ hot drinks.

3. When I'm hot and thirsty, I'd rather have a cold drink ___than___ a hot drink.

4. I prefer tea _____ coffee.

5. I like tea better _____ coffee.

6. I'd rather drink tea _____ coffee.

7. When I choose a movie to watch, I prefer comedies _____ drama.

8. I like folk music music better _____ rock and roll.

9. My parents would rather work _____ retire. They enjoy their jobs.

10. Do you like spring better _____ fall?

11. I prefer visiting my friends in the evening _____ watching TV by myself.

12. I would rather read a book in the evening _____ visit with friends.

EXERCISE 59 ▸ Let's talk: pairwork. (Chart 7-15)

Work with a partner. Take turns asking and answering questions. Be sure to answer in complete sentences.

Which do you like better?

Examples: Which do you prefer: apples or oranges?*
  → *I prefer oranges to apples.*

  Which do you like better: bananas or strawberries?
  → *I like bananas better than strawberries.*

  Which would you rather have right now: an apple or a banana?
  → *I'd rather have a banana.*

1. Which do you like better: rice or potatoes?
2. Which do you prefer: peas or corn?
3. Which would you rather have for dinner tonight: fish or chicken?
4. Name two sports. Which do you like better?
5. Name two movies. Which one would you rather see?
6. What kind of music would you rather listen to: rock or classical?
7. Name two vegetables. Which do you prefer?
8. Name two TV programs. Which do you like better?

EXERCISE 60 ▸ Let's talk: interview. (Chart 7-15)

Interview your classmates. Use ***would rather ... than*** in your answers. Share some of your answers with the class.

Would you rather ...

1. live in an apartment or in a house?** Why?
2. be an author or an artist? Why?
3. drive a fast car or fly a small plane? Why?
4. be rich and unlucky in love or poor and lucky in love? Why?
5. surf the internet or watch TV? Why?
6. have a big family or a small family? Why?
7. be a bird or a fish? Why?
8. spend your free time with other people or by yourself? Why?

---

*Use a rising intonation on the first choice and a falling intonation on the second choice: *Which do you prefer, apples or oranges?*

It is possible but not necessary to repeat a preposition after ***than*.
  CORRECT: *I'd rather live in an apartment **than in a house**.*
  CORRECT: *I'd rather live in an apartment **than a house**.*

7-16 Summary: Modal Auxiliaries Taught in Chapter 7

Auxiliary + the Simple Form of a Verb		Meaning
can	(a) Olga *can speak* English. (b) You *can go* now. (c) *Can* I *leave* early?	ability permission request
could	(d) He *couldn't come* to class. (e) It *could snow* tomorrow. (f) *Could* you *help* me?	past ability possibility request
may	(g) It *may rain* tomorrow. (h) You *may leave* now. (i) *May* I *see* your passport?	possibility permission request (with *I*, not *you*)
might	(j) It *might rain* tomorrow.	possibility
should	(k) Mary *should study* harder.	advice
had better	(l) I *had better study* tonight.	advice
must	(m) You *must register* by tomorrow (n) You worked all night. You *must be* tired.	necessity logical conclusion
will	(o) I *will be* in class tomorrow. (p) *Will* you *help* me carry this box?	certainty request
would	(q) *Would* you *help* me carry this box?	request (with *you*, not *I*)
Auxiliary + to + the Simple Form of a Verb		
have to	(r) I *have to study* tonight. (s) I *don't have to study* tonight. (t) I *didn't have to study* last night.	necessity lack of necessity (negative)
have got to	(u) I *have got to study* tonight.	necessity
be able to	(v) Kate *is able to study* today. (w) She *wasn't able to study* yesterday.	ability
ought to	(x) Kate *ought to study* harder.	advice

EXERCISE 61 ▸ Check your knowledge. (Chapter 7 Review)
Correct the errors.

    had
1. You ˄ better call the doctor today.

2. Emma shouldn't wears shorts to work.

3. Would you please to help me clean the kitchen?

4. George was able to talking by the age of one.

5. Today might a good day to go to the zoo with the kids.

6. I ought paying my bills today.

7. You don't should stay up too late tonight.

8. Can you speak any English a few years ago?

9. May you give me your name, please?

10. We must wait a long time for the subway last night.

11. You don't has to wait for me. I'll be a little late.

12. You won't tell anyone my secret, are you?

13. Please you unlock the door for me. I can't find my key.

14. Let's to take a break.

15. I prefer cooking vegetables to eat them raw.

EXERCISE 62 ▶ Reading, speaking, and writing. (Chapter 7)

Part I. Read the blog entry by co-author Stacy Hagen. Give the meaning for each of the boldfaced words. You can use Chart 7-16 for reference. Then find at least two uses of the imperative that give advice.

> Do you know these words?
> - impression   - prompt
> - formally   - résumé
> - suit   - discomfort
> - casual   - nervousness
> - value   - unprofessional

BlackBookBlog

How to Make a Good Impression in a Job Interview

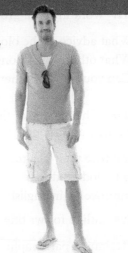

As you know, it is important to make a good impression when you interview for a job. For example, the way you dress can create a positive or negative impression. When I applied for my first job, many years ago, people dressed more formally. At the time, women wore dresses or skirts, never pants, and men wore suits. Now, you can be a little more casual. Sometimes women wear nice pants, and men **don't have to** always wear suits. It depends on the company you want to work for. Different companies have different work cultures.

However, there are certain things you **should** and **shouldn't** do to make a good impression. For example, you shouldn't wear flip-flops or shorts. This is probably too casual unless you are applying to be a surfing instructor!

> Are this man's clothes appropriate for a job interview? Why or why not?

Be sure to arrive on time or even a little early. Employers value workers who are prompt.

The interviewer will already have the résumé you sent, but you **might** want to bring extra copies. There **may** be more than one interviewer, and it's helpful if everyone has a copy of your résumé.

Greet the interviewer by name. Say, "Hello," or "Hi, Ms. Thompson*." It's common to follow with "It's nice to meet you." If you are in a culture where shaking hands is common, you can put out your hand at the same time. "Hey" is not an appropriate greeting and may create a negative impression. Save it for informal situations or for friends.

When you are answering the interviewer's questions, make eye contact. In many countries like the U.S. and Canada, this shows confidence and interest. Looking down or away may communicate discomfort or nervousness.

You probably already know this, but don't chew gum during the interview. It makes noise and looks unprofessional.

Finally, you will want to prepare for your interview. Look up common interview questions on the internet and practice answers. (There are many sites that give useful advice for different types of companies.) Also, you **ought to** research the company before you go to the interview. That way, you **can** show some knowledge of the company as you talk about the job. It can also help you think of good questions to ask. Often at the end of the interview, the interviewer asks if you have questions about the company.

If you follow these suggestions, you will have a better chance of making a good impression when you go for a job interview. Good luck!

*In formal situations, you can say, "How do you do?" instead of "Hello" or "Hi."

Part II. Work in small groups and discuss these questions.

1. What advice in the blog is the same as in your country and what advice is different?
2. What other suggestions can you think of to make a good impression at a job interview?
3. Can you think of other things a person in your country should never do at a job interview?

Part III. Choose one of the topics below. Write a three-paragraph blog entry of your own. Using Part I as a model, give general advice to people who want to …

1. improve their health.
2. get good grades.
3. improve their English.
4. find a job.
5. get a good night's sleep.
6. protect the environment by recycling.

Use this outline for writing your three paragraphs.

I. Beginning paragraph: *Do you want to … ? Here are some suggestions for you to consider.*
II. Middle paragraph: List your suggestions and add details, making use of modal verbs and the imperative.
III. Concluding paragraph: *Follow these suggestions for …*

An outline, formatted as shown below, is useful for organizing your writing.

Use roman numbers to show the topic of each paragraph. Use capital letters to show details under your topics.

    I. Introduction
   II. Suggestions
       A.
       B.
       C.
       etc.
  III. Conclusion

Part IV. Edit your writing. Check for the following:

1. ☐ use of your outline to guide your writing
2. ☐ correct use of different modal verbs or the imperative to give advice
3. ☐ use of *to* when necessary with the modal
4. ☐ no *-s* on the main verbs that come after modals
5. ☐ correct spelling (use a dictionary or spell-check)

▨▨▨▨▨ For digital resources, go to the Pearson Practice English app.

Appendix

Supplementary Grammar Charts

UNIT A

A-1 The Principal Parts of a Verb

Regular Verbs

SIMPLE FORM	SIMPLE PAST	PAST PARTICIPLE	PRESENT PARTICIPLE
call	called	called	calling
clean	cleaned	cleaned	cleaning
plan	planned	planned	planning
play	played	played	playing
try	tried	tried	trying

Irregular Verbs

SIMPLE FORM	SIMPLE PAST	PAST PARTICIPLE	PRESENT PARTICIPLE
eat	ate	eaten	eating
break	broke	broken	breaking
come	came	come	coming
sing	sang	sung	singing
put	put	put	putting

Principal Parts of a Verb

(1)	THE SIMPLE FORM	English verbs have four principal forms, or "parts." *The simple form* is the form that is found in a dictionary. It is the base form with no endings on it (no final **-s**, **-ed**, or **-ing**).
(2)	THE SIMPLE PAST	*The simple past* ends in **-ed** for regular verbs. Most verbs are regular, but many common verbs have irregular past forms.
(3)	THE PAST PARTICIPLE	*The past participle* also ends in **-ed** for regular verbs. Other verbs have irregular past participles. Past participles are used with the perfect tenses (Chapter 4) and the passive (Chapter 10).
(4)	THE PRESENT PARTICIPLE	*The present participle* ends in **-ing** (for both regular and irregular verbs). It is used in progressive tenses (e.g., the present progressive and the past progressive).

The woman *is calling* for help again. Her car *broke* down in the snow. She *called* for a tow truck an hour ago, but no one *has come* yet.

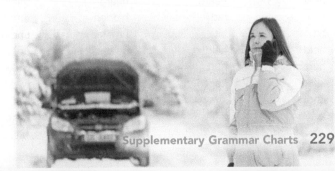

A-2 Common Irregular Verbs: A Reference List

SIMPLE FORM	SIMPLE PAST	PAST PARTICIPLE	SIMPLE FORM	SIMPLE PAST	PAST PARTICIPLE
be	was, were	been	lend	lent	lent
beat	beat	beaten	let	let	let
become	became	become	lie	lay	lain
begin	began	begun	light	lit/lighted	lit/lighted
bend	bent	bent	lose	lost	lost
bite	bit	bitten	make	made	made
blow	blew	blown	mean	meant	meant
break	broke	broken	meet	met	met
bring	brought	brought	pay	paid	paid
build	built	built	put	put	put
burn	burned/burnt	burned/burnt	quit	quit	quit
buy	bought	bought	read	read	read
catch	caught	caught	ride	rode	ridden
choose	chose	chosen	ring	rang	rung
come	came	come	rise	rose	risen
cost	cost	cost	run	ran	run
cut	cut	cut	say	said	said
dig	dug	dug	see	saw	seen
do	did	done	sell	sold	sold
draw	drew	drawn	send	sent	sent
dream	dreamed/dreamt	dreamed/dreamt	set	set	set
drink	drank	drunk	shake	shook	shaken
drive	drove	driven	shoot	shot	shot
eat	ate	eaten	shut	shut	shut
fall	fell	fallen	sing	sang	sung
feed	fed	fed	sink	sank	sunk
feel	felt	felt	sit	sat	sat
fight	fought	fought	sleep	slept	slept
find	found	found	slide	slid	slid
fit	fit	fit	speak	spoke	spoken
fly	flew	flown	spend	spent	spent
forget	forgot	forgotten	spread	spread	spread
forgive	forgave	forgiven	stand	stood	stood
freeze	froze	frozen	steal	stole	stolen
get	got	got/gotten	stick	stuck	stuck
give	gave	given	swim	swam	swum
go	went	gone	take	took	taken
grow	grew	grown	teach	taught	taught
hang	hung	hung	tear	tore	torn
have	had	had	tell	told	told
hear	heard	heard	think	thought	thought
hide	hid	hidden	throw	threw	thrown
hit	hit	hit	understand	understood	understood
hold	held	held	upset	upset	upset
hurt	hurt	hurt	wake	woke/waked	woken/waked
keep	kept	kept	wear	wore	worn
know	knew	known	win	won	won
leave	left	left	write	wrote	written

A-3 The Present Perfect vs. The Past Perfect

PRESENT PERFECT before now / now	(a) I am not hungry now. I *have* already *eaten*.	The PRESENT PERFECT expresses an activity that *occurred before now*, at *an unspecified time in the past,* as in (a).
PAST PERFECT before 1:00 / 1:00 P.M.	(b) I was not hungry at 1:00 P.M. I *had* already *eaten*.	The PAST PERFECT expresses an activity that *occurred before **another** time in the past*. In (b): I ate at noon. I was not hungry at 1:00 P.M. because I had already eaten before 1:00 P.M.

A-4 The Past Progressive vs. The Past Perfect

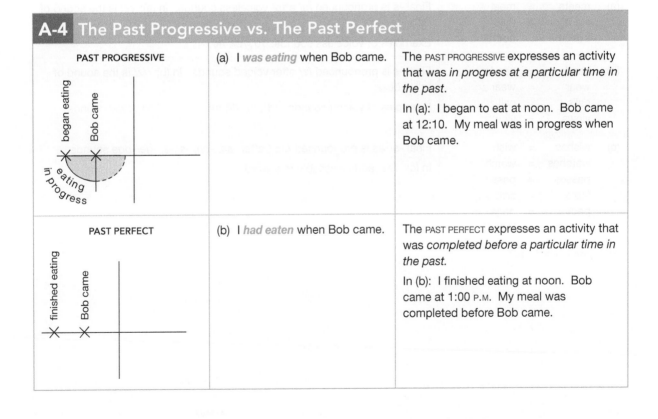

PAST PROGRESSIVE began eating / Bob came / eating in progress	(a) I *was eating* when Bob came.	The PAST PROGRESSIVE expresses an activity that was *in progress at a particular time in the past*. In (a): I began to eat at noon. Bob came at 12:10. My meal was in progress when Bob came.
PAST PERFECT finished eating / Bob came	(b) I *had eaten* when Bob came.	The PAST PERFECT expresses an activity that was *completed before a particular time in the past*. In (b): I finished eating at noon. Bob came at 1:00 P.M. My meal was completed before Bob came.

A-5 Regular Verbs: Pronunciation of -ed Endings

(a) talked	=	talk/t/
stopped	=	stop/t/
missed	=	miss/t/
watched	=	watch/t/
washed	=	wash/t/

Final **-ed** is pronounced /t/ after voiceless sounds.
You make a voiceless sound by pushing air through your mouth.
No sound comes from your throat.

Examples of voiceless sounds: /k/, /p/, /s/, /ch/, /sh/.

(b) called	=	call/d/
rained	=	rain/d/
lived	=	live/d/
robbed	=	rob/d/
stayed	=	stay/d/

Final **-ed** is pronounced /d/ after voiced sounds.
You make a voiced sound from your throat. Your voice box vibrates.

Examples of voiced sounds: /l/, /n/, /v/, /b/, and all vowel sounds.

(c) waited	=	wait/əd/
needed	=	need/əd/

Final **-ed** is pronounced /əd/* after "t" and "d" sounds.

In (c): /əd/ adds a syllable to a word.

*/əd/ is pronounced "ud."

A-6 Pronunciation of Final -s/-es for Verbs and Nouns

Final **-s/-es** on verbs and nouns has three different pronunciations: /s/, /z/, and /əz/.

(a)	meets	=	meet/s/
	helps	=	help/s/
	books	=	book/s/

Final **-s** is pronounced /s/ after voiceless sounds. In (a): /s/ is the sound of "s" in bus.

Examples of voiceless sounds: /t/, /p/, /k/.

(b)	needs	=	need/z/
	wear	=	wear/z/
	calls	=	call/z/
	views	=	view/z/

Final **-s** is pronounced /z/ after voiced sounds. In (b): /z/ is the sound of "z" in buzz.

Examples of voiced sounds: /d/, /r/, /l/, /m/, /b/, and all vowel sounds.

(c)	wishes	=	wish/əz/
	watches	=	watch/əz/
	passes	=	pass/əz/
	sizes	=	size/əz/
	pages	=	page/əz/
	judges	=	judge/əz/

Final **-s/-es** is pronounced /əz/* after -sh, -ch, -s, -z, -ge/-dge sounds.

In (c): /əz/ adds a syllable to a word.

*/əz/ is pronounced "uz."

A-7 Review: Subject and Object Pronouns, Possessive Pronouns, and Possessive Adjectives

SUBJECT PRONOUNS	OBJECT PRONOUNS	POSSESSIVE PRONOUNS	POSSESSIVE ADJECTIVES
I	me	mine	**my** name(s)
you	you	yours	**your** name(s)
she	her	hers	**her** name(s)
he	him	his	**his** name(s)
it	it	its	**its** name(s)
we	us	ours	**our** name(s)
you	you	yours	**your** name(s)
they	them	theirs	**their** name(s)

(a) *We* saw an accident.	Personal pronouns are used as:
(b) Sonya saw *it* too.	• subjects, as in (a);
(c) I have my pen. Ella has *hers*.	• objects, as in (b); OR
(d) *Her* pen is blue.	• to show possession, as in (c)
	Possessive adjectives also show possession, as in (d).

(e) I have a *book*. *It* is on my desk.	Use a singular pronoun to refer to a singular noun. In (e): *book* and *it* are both singular.
(f) I have some *books*. *They* are on my desk.	Use a plural pronoun to refer to a plural noun. In (f): *books* and *they* are both plural.

(g) *It's* sunny today.	COMPARE: In (g): ***it's*** = *it is*
(h) I'm studying about India. I'm interested in *its* history.	In (h): ***its*** is a possessive adjective: *its history* = *India's history*
INCORRECT: *I'm interested in it's history.*	A possessive adjective has NO apostrophe.

A-8 Comparison of *Yes/No* and Information Question Forms

(Question Word)	Helping Verb	Subject	Main Verb	(Rest of Sentence)	
(a)	*Does*	Leo	*live*	in Montreal?	
(b) Where	*does*	Leo	*live*?		
(c)	*Is*	Sara	*studying*	at the library?	
(d) Where	*is*	Sara	*studying*?		
(e)	*Will*	you	*help*	me?	
(f) When	*will*	you	*help*	me?	
(g)	*Did*	they	*see*	Mario?	
(h) Who(m)	*did*	they	*see*?		
(i)	*Is*	Olaf	at home?		
(j) Where	*is*	Olaf?			
(k)		*Who*	*came*?		When the question word (e.g., ***who*** or ***what***) is the subject of the sentence, ***do*** or ***does*** is never used.
(l)		*What*	*happened*?		

UNIT B: Phrasal Verbs

NOTE: See the *Fundamentals of English Grammar Workbook* appendix for practice exercises for phrasal verbs.

B-1 Phrasal Verbs

(a) We *put off* our trip. We'll go next month instead of this month. (*put off = postpone*)	In (a): ***put off*** = a phrasal verb
	A PHRASAL VERB = a verb and a particle that together have a special meaning. For example, *put off* means "postpone."
(b) Jimmy, *put on* your coat before you go outdoors. (*put on = place clothes on one's body*)	A PARTICLE = a "small word" (e.g., *off, on, away, back*) that is used in a phrasal verb.
(c) Someone left the scissors on the table. They didn't belong there. I *put* them *away*. (*put away = put something in its usual or proper place*)	Note that the phrasal verbs with ***put*** in (a), (b), (c), and (d) all have different meanings.
(d) After I used the dictionary, I *put* it *back* on the shelf. (*put back = return something to its original place*)	

Separable

	Some phrasal verbs are **separable**: A NOUN OBJECT can either
(e) We *put off our trip*. = (VERB + **particle** + NOUN)	(1) follow the particle, as in (e), OR
(f) We *put our trip off*. = (VERB + NOUN + **particle**)	(2) come between (separate) the verb and the particle, as in (f).
(g) We *put it off*. = (VERB + PRONOUN + **particle**)	If a phrasal verb is separable, a PRONOUN OBJECT comes between the verb and the particle, as in (g).
	INCORRECT: We put off it.

Nonseparable

	If a phrasal verb is **nonseparable**, a NOUN or PRONOUN always follows (never precedes) the particle, as in (h) and (i).
(h) I *ran into Bob*. = (VERB + **particle** + NOUN)	
(i) I *ran into him*. = (VERB + **particle** + PRONOUN)	*INCORRECT: I ran Bob into.*
	INCORRECT: I ran him into.

Phrasal Verbs: Intransitive

	Some phrasal verbs are intransitive; i.e., they are not followed by an object.
(j) The machine *broke down*.	
(k) Please *come in*.	
(l) Mr. Lim *passed away*.	

Three-Word Phrasal Verbs

(m) Last night some friends *dropped in*.	Some two-word verbs (e.g., *drop in*) can become three-word verbs (e.g., *drop in on*).
	In (m): ***drop in*** is not followed by an object. It is an intransitive phrasal verb (i.e., it is not followed by an object).
(n) Let's *drop in on* Alice this afternoon.	In (n): ***drop in on*** is a three-word phrasal verb. Three-word phrasal verbs are transitive (they are followed by objects).
(o) We *dropped in on her* last week.	In (o): Three-word phrasal verbs are nonseparable (the noun or pronoun follows the phrasal verb).

A ask out = ask (someone) to go on a date

B blow out = extinguish (a match, a candle)
break down = stop functioning properly
break out = happen suddenly
break up = separate, end a relationship
bring back = return
bring up = (1) raise (children)
　　　　　　 (2) mention, start to talk about

C call back = return a telephone call
call off = cancel
call on = ask (someone) to speak in class
call up = make a telephone call
cheer up = make happier
clean up = make neat and clean
come along (with) = accompany
come from = originate
come in = enter a room or building
come over (to) = visit the speaker's place
cross out = draw a line through
cut out (of) = remove with scissors or knife

D dress up = put on nice clothes
drop in (on) = visit without calling first or
　　　　　　 without an invitation
drop out (of) = stop attending (school)

E eat out = eat at a restaurant

F fall down = fall to the ground
figure out = find the solution to a problem
fill in = complete by writing in a blank space
fill out = write information on a form
fill up = fill completely with gas, water, coffee,
　　　　　　 etc.
find out (about) = discover information
fool around (with) = have fun while wasting
　　　　　　　　　 time

G get on = enter a bus/an airplane/a train/a
　　　　　　 subway
get out of = leave a car, a taxi

get over = recover from an illness or a shock
get together (with) = join, meet
get through (with) = finish
get up = get out of bed in the morning
give away = donate, get rid of by giving
give back = return (something) to (someone)
give up = quit doing (something) or quit trying
go on = continue
go back (to) = return to a place
go out = not stay home
go over (to) = (1) approach
　　　　　　 (2) visit another's home
grow up (in) = become an adult

H hand in = give homework, test papers, etc., to a
　　　　　　 teacher
hand out = give (something) to this person,
　　　　　　 then to that person, then to
　　　　　　 another person, etc.
hang around/out (with) = spend time relaxing
hang up = (1) hang on a hanger or a hook
　　　　　　 (2) end a telephone conversation
have on = wear
help out = assist (someone)

K keep away (from) = not give to
keep on = continue

L lay off = stop employment
leave on = (1) not turn off (a light, a machine)
　　　　　　 (2) not take off (clothing)
look into = investigate
look over = examine carefully
look out (for) = be careful
look up = look for information in a dictionary,
　　　　　　 a telephone directory, an
　　　　　　 encyclopedia, etc.

P pay back = return borrowed money to (someone)
pick up = lift
point out = call attention to

(continued)

print out = create a paper copy from a computer

put away = put (something) in its usual or proper place

put back = return (something) to its original place

put down = stop holding or carrying

put off = postpone

put on = put clothes on one's body

put out = extinguish (stop) a fire, a cigarette

R **run into** = meet by chance

run out (of) = finish the supply of (something)

S **set out (for)** = begin a trip

shut off = stop a machine or a light, turn off

sign up (for) = put one's name on a list

show up = come, appear

sit around (with) = sit and do nothing

sit back = put one's back against a chair back

sit down = go from standing to sitting

speak up = speak louder

stand up = go from sitting to standing

start over = begin again

stay up = not go to bed

T **take back** = return

take off = (1) remove clothes from one's body
(2) ascend in an airplane

take out = invite out and pay

talk over = discuss

tear down = destroy a building

tear out (of) = remove (paper) by tearing

tear up = tear into small pieces

think over = consider

throw away/out = put in the trash, discard

try on = put on clothing to see if it fits

turn around ⎫
turn back ⎬ change to the opposite direction

turn down = decrease the volume

turn off = stop a machine or a light

turn on = start a machine or a light

turn over = turn the top side to the bottom

turn up = increase the volume

W **wake up** = stop sleeping

watch out (for) = be careful

work out = solve

write down = write a note on a piece of paper

UNIT C: Prepositions

NOTE: See the *Fundamentals of English Grammar Workbook* appendix for practice exercises for preposition combinations.

C-1 Preposition Combinations: Introduction

ADJ + PREP (a) Ali is *absent from* class today. V + PREP (b) This book *belongs to* me.	*At, from, of, on,* and *to* are examples of prepositions. Prepositions are often combined with adjectives, as in (a), and verbs, as in (b).

C-2 Preposition Combinations: A Reference List

A
be absent from
be accustomed to
   add (*this*) to (*that*)
be acquainted with
   admire (*someone*) for (*something*)
be afraid of
   agree with (*someone*) about (*something*)
be angry at / with (*someone*) about / over (*something*)
   apologize to (*someone*) for (*something*)
   apply for (*something*)
   approve of
   argue with (*someone*) about / over (*something*)
   arrive at (*a building / a room*)
   arrive in (*a city / a country*)
   ask (*someone*) about (*something*)
   ask (*someone*) for (*something*)
be aware of

B
be bad for
   believe in
   belong to
be bored with / by
   borrow (*something*) from (*someone*)

C
be clear to
   combine with
   compare (*this*) to / with (*that*)
   complain to (*someone*) about (*something*)
be composed of
   concentrate on
   consist of
be crazy about
be crowded with
be curious about

D
   depend on (*someone*) for (*something*)
be dependent on (*someone*) for (*something*)

be devoted to
   die of / from
be different from
   disagree with (*someone*) about (*something*)
be disappointed in
   discuss (*something*) with (*someone*)
   divide (*this*) into (*that*)
be divorced from
be done with
   dream about / of
   dream of

E
be engaged to
be equal to
   escape from (*a place*)
be excited about
   excuse (*someone*) for (*something*)
   excuse from
be exhausted from

F
be familiar with
be famous for
   feel about
   feel like
   fill (*something*) with
be finished with
   forgive (*someone*) for (*something*)
be friendly to / with
be frightened of / by
be full of

G
   get rid of
be gone from
be good for
   graduate from

(continued)

H
happen to
be happy about (*something*)
be happy for (*someone*)
hear about / of (*something*) from (*someone*)
help (*someone*) with (*something*)
hide (*something*) from (*someone*)
hope for
be hungry for

I
insist on
be interested in
introduce (*someone*) to (*someone*)
invite (*someone*) to (*something*)
be involved in

K
be kind to
know about

L
laugh at
leave for (a *place*)
listen to
look at
look for
look forward to
look like

M
be made of
be married to
matter to
be the matter with
multiply (*this*) by (*that*)

N
be nervous about
be nice to

O
be opposed to

P
pay for
be patient with
be pleased with / about
play with
point at
be polite to
prefer (*this*) to (*that*)

be prepared for
protect (*this*) from (*that*)
be proud of
provide (*someone*) with

Q
be qualified for

R
read about
be ready for
be related to
rely on
be responsible for

S
be sad about
be satisfied with
be scared of / by
search for
separate (*this*) from (*that*)
be similar to
speak to / with (*someone*) about (*something*)
stare at
subtract (*this*) from (*that*)
be sure of / about

T
take care of
talk about (*something*)
talk to / with (*someone*) about (*something*)
tell (*someone*) about (*something*)
be terrified of / by
thank (*someone*) for (*something*)
think about / of
be thirsty for
be tired from
be tired of
translate from (*one language*) to (*another*)

U
be used to

W
wait for
wait on
warn about / of
wave at
wonder about
be worried about

Listening Script

EXERCISE 1 ▸ p. xiii.

Part I

It's Nice to Meet You

DANIEL:	Hi. My name is Daniel.
SOFIA:	Hi. I'm Sofia. It's nice to meet you.
DANIEL:	Nice to meet you too. Where are you from?
SOFIA:	I'm from Montreal. How about you?
DANIEL:	I'm from Miami.
SOFIA:	Are you a new student?
DANIEL:	Yes, and no. This is my third year of college, but I'm new here.
SOFIA:	This is my second year here. I'm in the business school. I really like it.
DANIEL:	Oh, my major is economics! Maybe we'll have a class together. So, tell me a little more about yourself. What do you like to do in your free time?
SOFIA:	I love the outdoors. I spend a lot of time in the mountains. I hike on weekends. I write about it on social media.
DANIEL:	I spend a lot of time outdoors too. I like the beach. In the summer, I swim every day.
SOFIA:	This town has a great beach.
DANIEL:	Yeah, I want to go there! Now, when I introduce you to the group, I have to write your full name on the board. What's your last name, and how do you spell it?
SOFIA:	It's Sanchez. S-A-N-C-H-E-Z.
DANIEL:	My last name is Willson — with two "l"s: W-I-L-L-S-O-N.
SOFIA:	Oh, it looks like our time is up. I enjoyed our conversation.
DANIEL:	Thanks. I enjoyed it too.

Chapter 1: Present Time

EXERCISE 9 ▸ p. 7.

1. Irene designs video games.
2. She is working on a new project.
3. She is sitting in front of her computer.
4. She spends her weekends at the office.
5. She's finishing plans for a new game.

EXERCISE 10 ▸ p. 8.

A Problem with the Printer

1. Does it need more paper?
2. Does it have enough ink?
3. Are you fixing it yourself?
4. Do you know how to fix it?
5. Do we have another printer in the office?
6. Hmmm. Is it my imagination, or is it making a strange noise?

EXERCISE 14 ▸ p. 10.

Natural Disasters: A Flood

1. The weather causes some natural disasters.
2. Heavy rains sometimes create floods.
3. A big flood causes a lot of damage.
4. In towns, floods can damage buildings, homes, and roads.
5. After a flood, a town needs a lot of financial help for repairs.

EXERCISE 18 ▸ p. 12.

1. talks	9. mixes
2. fishes	10. watches
3. hopes	11. studies
4. teaches	12. buys
5. moves	13. enjoys
6. kisses	14. tries
7. pushes	15. carries
8. waits	

EXERCISE 37 ▸ p. 24.

Part II

1. Do you have pain anywhere?
2. Does it hurt anywhere else?
3. Does she have a cough or sore throat?
4. Does he have a fever?
5. Does she need lab tests?
6. Am I very sick?
7. Is it serious?
8. Does he need to make another appointment?
9. Do they want to wait in the waiting room?
10. Do we pay now or later?

EXERCISE 39 ▶ p. 25.

Getting Ready to Leave

1. We have a few minutes before we need to leave.
   Do you want a cup of coffee?
2. I'm ready. Do you need help?
3. Look outside. Is it raining hard?
4. Do we need to take an umbrella?
5. Mr. Smith has his coat on. Is he leaving now?
6. I'm looking for the elevators. Are they near here?

EXERCISE 41 ▶ p. 28.

Part III

Many people do aerobic exercise. It is a special type of exercise. Aerobic exercise makes the heart beat fast. Running, fast walking, and dancing are some examples of this exercise.

Right now some people are exercising in an exercise class. They are listening to music, and they are dancing. Their hearts are beating fast. Many parts of their body are getting exercise.

How about you? Do you exercise every day? Do you do aerobic exercise?

Chapter 2: Past Time

EXERCISE 17 ▶ p. 40.

1. watch, watched
2. called, called
3. works, worked
4. decided, decided

EXERCISE 18 ▶ p. 41.

In the Classroom

1. The teacher explains the homework …
2. The teacher explained the homework …
3. We review new vocabulary …
4. Our teacher surprised us …
5. My friend practices pronunciation …
6. We watched an interesting video …
7. We started a project …
8. We finish a chapter …

EXERCISE 19 ▶ p. 41.

Part II

1. Alex hurt his finger. Did he cut it with a knife?
2. Ms. Jones doesn't have any money in her wallet. Did she spend it all yesterday?
3. Karen's parents visited. Did you meet them yesterday?
4. The Browns don't have a car anymore. Did they sell it?
5. I dropped the glass. Did I break it?
6. Ann didn't throw away her old clothes. Did she keep them?
7. John gave a book to his son. Did he read it to him?
8. You don't have your glasses. Did you lose them?
9. Mr. Jones looked for his passport in his desk drawer. Did he find it?
10. The baby is crying. Did I upset her?

EXERCISE 20 ▶ p. 42.

Part II

At a Wedding

1. The bride wasn't nervous before the ceremony.
2. The groom was nervous before the ceremony.
3. His parents weren't nervous about the wedding.
4. The bride and groom were excited about their wedding.
5. The ceremony was in the evening.
6. The wedding reception wasn't after the wedding.
7. It was the next day.
8. It was at a popular hotel.
9. A lot of guests were there.
10. Some relatives from out of town weren't there.

EXERCISE 25 ▶ p. 45.

Part I

A: Did you have a good weekend?
B: Yeah, I went to a waterslide park.
A: Really? That sounds like fun!
B: It was great! I loved the fast slides. How about you? How was your weekend?
A: I visited my aunt.
B: Did you have a good time?
A: Not really. She didn't like my clothes or my haircut.

EXERCISE 40 ▶ p. 55.

Jennifer's Problem

Jennifer works for an insurance company. When people need help with their car insurance, they call her. Right now it is 9:05 a.m., and Jennifer is working at her desk.

She came to work on time this morning. Yesterday Jennifer was late to work because she had a car accident. While she was driving to work, her cell phone rang. She reached for it. While she was reaching for her phone, Jennifer lost control of the car. It hit a telephone pole.

Jennifer is OK now, but her car isn't. She feels very embarrassed. She made a bad decision, especially since it is illegal to talk on a cell phone and drive at the same time in her city.

EXERCISE 41 ▶ p. 56.

At a Checkout Stand in a Grocery Store

1. CASHIER: Hi. Did you find what you needed?
   CUSTOMER: Almost everything. I was looking for sticky rice, but I didn't see it.
   CASHIER: It's on aisle 10, in the Asian food section.
2. CASHIER: This is the express lane. Ten items only. It looks like you have more than ten. Did you count them?
   CUSTOMER: I thought I had ten. Oh, I guess I have more. Sorry.
   CASHIER: The checkout stand next to me is open.

3. CASHIER: Do you have any coupons you wanted to use?
   CUSTOMER: I had a couple in my purse, but I can't find them now.
   CASHIER: What were they for? I might have some extras here.
   CUSTOMER: One was for eggs, and the other was for ice cream.
   CASHIER: I think I have those.

Chapter 3: Future Time

EXERCISE 13 ▶ p. 70.

A: Are you going to come with us to the meeting?
B: No, I'm going to study. I have a test tomorrow.
A: I understand. I'll let you know what happens.

EXERCISE 14 ▶ p. 71.

Part II
A: Where are you going to move to?
B: We're going to look for something outside the city. We're going to spend the weekend apartment hunting.
A: What fees are you going to need to pay?
B: I think we are going to need to pay the first and last month's rent.
A: Are there going to be other fees?
B: There is probably going to be an application fee and a cleaning fee. Also, the landlord is probably going to check our credit, so we are going to need to pay for that.

EXERCISE 15 ▶ p. 72.

Before the Party

1. We'll need to get the house ready for the party tomorrow, but I'll be gone in the morning.
2. You'll need to fold the laundry and dust the furniture.
3. I talked to your sister. She'll clean the kitchen.
4. Your dad will be home. He'll vacuum the carpets.
5. Your brothers won't be home. They'll do the cleanup.
6. Some of the guests are going to come early. We'll need to be ready by 5:00.

EXERCISE 16 ▶ p. 72.

Part II
At the Pharmacy

1. Your prescription'll be ready in ten minutes.
2. The medicine'll make you feel a little tired.
3. The pharmacist'll call your doctor's office.
4. This cough syrup'll help your cough.
5. Two aspirin'll be enough.
6. The generic drug'll cost less.
7. This information'll explain all the side effects for this medicine.

EXERCISE 25 ▶ p. 78.

My Day Tomorrow

1. It's going to snow. I need to find my warm clothes.
2. I'll probably do a few errands.
3. I may stop at the post office.
4. I will probably pick up groceries at the store.
5. The roads are going to be icy.
6. Maybe I'll do my errands midday.

EXERCISE 37 ▶ p. 84.

Going on Vacation

A: I'm going on vacation tomorrow.
B: Where are you going?
A: To San Francisco.
B: How are you getting there? Are you flying or driving your car?
A: I'm flying. I want to be at the airport by 7:00 tomorrow morning.
B: Do you need a ride to the airport?
A: No, thanks. I'm taking a taxi. What about you? Are you planning to go somewhere over vacation?
B: No. I'm staying here.

EXERCISE 46 ▶ p. 89.

At a Chinese Restaurant

A: OK, let's all open our fortune cookies.
B: What does your cookie say?
A: Mine says, "You will receive an unexpected gift." Great! Are you planning to give me a gift soon?
B: Not that I know of. Mine says, "Your life will be long and happy." Good. I want a long life.
C: Mine says, "A smile solves all communication problems." Well, that's good! After this, when I don't understand someone, I'll just smile at them.
D: My fortune is this: "If you work hard, you will be successful."
A: Well, it looks like all of us will have good luck in the future!

Chapter 4: Present Perfect and Past Perfect

EXERCISE 12 ▶ p. 98.

At a Restaurant

1. My coffee's a little cold already.
2. My coffee's gotten a little cold already.
3. Your order's not ready yet.
4. Wow! Our order's here already.
5. Excuse me, I think our waiter's forgotten our order.
6. Actually, your waiter's just gone home sick. I'll take care of you.

EXERCISE 22 ▶ p. 104.

Part II

1. The cash machine's been out of service for two days.
2. I'm sorry. You credit card's expired.

3. My checking account fees've increased a lot.
4. Someone's withdrawn money from your account.
5. Our new debit cards've gotten lost in the mail.

EXERCISE 28 ▶ p. 107.

1. Every day, I spend some money. Yesterday, I spent some money. Since Friday, I have ...
2. I usually make a big breakfast. Yesterday, I made a big breakfast. All week, I have ...
3. Every day, I send emails. Yesterday I sent an email. Today I have already ...
4. Every time I go to a restaurant, I leave a nice tip. Last night I left a nice tip. I just finished dinner, and I have ...
5. Every weekend, I sleep in late. Last weekend, I slept in late. Since I was a teenager, I have ...
6. I drive very carefully. On my last trip across the country, I drove very carefully. All my life, I have ...
7. Every morning, I sing in the shower. Earlier today, I sang in the shower. Since I was little, I have ...

EXERCISE 37 ▶ p. 112.

Today's Weather

The weather has certainly been changing today. Boy, what a day! We've already had rain, wind, hail, and sun. So, what's in store for tonight? As you have probably seen, dark clouds have been building. We have a weather system moving in that is going to bring colder temperatures and high winds. We've been saying all week that this system is coming, and it looks like tonight is it! We've even seen snow down south of us, and we could get some snow here too. So hang onto your hats! We may have a rough night ahead of us.

EXERCISE 39 ▶ p. 114.

1. A: What song is playing on the radio?
   B: I don't know, but it's good, isn't it?
2. A: How long have you lived in Dubai?
   B: About a year.
3. A: Where are the kids?
   B: I don't know. I've been calling them since I got home.
4. A: Who have you met tonight?
   B: Actually, I've met a few people from your office. How about you? Who have you met?
   A: I've met some interesting business people.

Chapter 5: Asking Questions

EXERCISE 6 ▶ p. 124.
Part II

At the Grocery Store

1. I need to see the manager. Is she available?
2. I need to see the manager. Is he in the store today?
3. Here is one bag of apples. Is that enough?
4. I need a drink of water. Is there a drinking fountain?
5. My credit card isn't working. Hmmm. Did it expire?

6. Where's Simon? Has he left?
7. The price seems high. Does it include the tax?

EXERCISE 11 ▶ p. 127.

A: Do you know Roberto and Isabelle?
B: Yes, I do. They live around the corner from me.
A: Have you seen them recently?
B: No, I haven't. They're out of town.
A: When are they going to be back? I'm having a party, and I can't reach them.
B: They're going to be back Monday. They are with Roberto's parents.
A: Oh, why are they there?
B: Because his dad is sick.
A: That's too bad.
B: Do you want Roberto's or Isabelle's cell number?
A: No, I don't, but thanks. I'll talk to them when they get back.
B: OK, sounds good.

EXERCISE 12 ▶ p. 127.

1. Do you want to go to the mall?
2. When are the Waltons coming?
3. Where will I meet you?
4. Why were you late?
5. What are you cleaning for?

EXERCISE 18 ▶ p. 130.

A Secret

A: John told me something.
B: What did he tell you?
A: It's confidential. I can't tell you.
B: Did he tell anyone else?
A: He told a few other people.
B: Who did he tell?
A: Some friends.
B: Then it's not a secret. What did he say?
A: I can't tell you.
B: Why can't you tell me?
A: Because it's about you. But don't worry. It's nothing bad.
B: Gee. Thanks a lot. That sure makes me feel better.

EXERCISE 29 ▶ p. 137.

1. A: How fresh are these eggs?
   B: I just bought them at the farmers' market, so they should be fine.
2. A: How cheap were the tickets?
   B: They were 50% off.
3. A: How hard was the driver's test?
   B: Well, I didn't pass, so that gives you an idea.
4. A: How clean is the car?
   B: There's dirt on the floor. We need to vacuum it inside.
5. A: How hot is the frying pan?
   B: Don't touch it! You'll burn yourself.
6. A: How noisy is the street you live on?
   B: There is a lot of traffic, so we keep the windows closed a lot.

7. A: How serious are you about interviewing for the job?
   B: Very. I already scheduled an interview with the company.

EXERCISE 33 ▶ p. 139.

Questions:
1. How old are you?
2. How tall are you?
3. How much do you weigh?
4. In general, how well do you sleep at night?
5. How quickly do you fall asleep?
6. How often do you wake up during the night?
7. How tired are you in the mornings?
8. How many times a week do you exercise?
9. How are you feeling right now?
10. How soon can you come in for an overnight appointment?

EXERCISE 41 ▶ p. 144.

1. Where's my key?
2. Where're my keys?
3. Who're those people?
4. What's in that box?
5. What're you doing?
6. Where'd Bob go last night?
7. Who'll be at the party?
8. Why's the teacher absent?
9. Who's that?
10. Why'd you say that?
11. Who'd you talk to at the party?
12. How're we going to get to work?
13. What'd you say?
14. How'll you do that?

EXERCISE 43 ▶ p. 145.

A Mother Talking to Her Teenage Daughter
1. Where're you going?
2. Who're you going with?
3. Who's that?
4. How long've you known him?
5. Where'd you meet him?
6. Where's he go to school?
7. Is he a good student?
8. What time'll you be back?
9. Why're you wearing that outfit?
10. Why're you giving me that look?
11. Why am I asking so many questions? Because I love you!

EXERCISE 44 ▶ p. 145.

1. What do you (*Whaddaya*) want to do?
2. What are you (*Whaddaya*) doing?
3. What are you (*Whaddaya*) having for dinner?
4. What are you (*Whaddaya*) doing that for?
5. What do you (*Whaddaya*) think about that?
6. What are you (*Whaddaya*) laughing for?
7. What do you (*Whaddaya*) need?
8. What do you (*Whaddaya*) have in your pocket?

EXERCISE 50 ▶ p. 148.

1. A: Did you like the movie?
   B: It was OK, I guess. How about you?
   A: I thought it was pretty good.
2. A: Are you going to the company party?
   B: I haven't decided yet. What about you?
   A: I think I will.
3. A: Do you like living in this city?
   B: Sort of. How about you?
   A: I'm not sure. It's pretty noisy.
4. A: What are you going to have?
   B: Well, I'm not really hungry. I think I might just order a salad. How about you?
   A: I'll have one too.

EXERCISE 54 ▶ p. 150.

1. Simple Present
   a. You like strong coffee, don't you?
   b. David goes to Ames High School, doesn't he?
   c. Leila and Sara live on Tree Road, don't they?
   d. Jane has the keys to the storeroom, doesn't she?
   e. Jane's in her office, isn't she?
   f. You're a member of this class, aren't you?
   g. Oleg doesn't have a car, does he?
   h. Lisa isn't from around here, is she?
   i. I'm in trouble, aren't I?
2. Simple Past
   a. Paul went to Indonesia, didn't he?
   b. You didn't talk to the boss, did you?
   c. Ted's parents weren't at home, were they?
   d. That was Pat's idea, wasn't it?
3. Present Progressive, *Be Going To,* and Past Progressive
   a. You're studying hard, aren't you?
   b. Greg isn't working at the bank, is he?
   c. It isn't going to rain today, is it?
   d. Michelle and Yoko were helping, weren't they?
   e. He wasn't listening, was he?
4. Present Perfect
   a. It has been warmer than usual, hasn't it?
   b. You've had a lot of homework, haven't you?
   c. We haven't spent much time together, have we?
   d. Fatima has started her new job, hasn't she?
   e. Bruno hasn't finished his sales report yet, has he?
   f. Steve's had to leave early, hasn't he?

EXERCISE 56, p. 151.

Checking in at a Hotel
1. You have our reservation, don't you?
2. We have a non-smoking room, don't we?
3. There's a view of the city, isn't there?
4. I didn't give you my credit card yet, did I?
5. The room rate doesn't include tax, does it?
6. The price includes breakfast, right?
7. Check-out time isn't until noon, is it?
8. There are hair dryers in the rooms, aren't there?
9. You don't have a pool, do you?
10. There isn't a hot tub, is there?

EXERCISE 58 ▶ p. 153.

Part I

Ordering at a Fast-Food Restaurant

CASHIER: So, what'll it be?
CUSTOMER: I'll have a burger.
CASHIER: Would you like fries or a salad with your burger?
CUSTOMER: I'll have fries.
CASHIER: What size?
CUSTOMER: Medium.
CASHIER: Anything to drink?
CUSTOMER: I'll have a vanilla shake.
CASHIER: Size?
CUSTOMER: Medium.
CASHIER: OK. So that's a burger, fries, vanilla shake.
CUSTOMER: About how long'll it take?
CASHIER: We're pretty crowded right now. Probably 10 minutes or so. That'll be $6.50. Your number's on the receipt. I'll call the number when your order's ready.
CUSTOMER: Thanks.

Chapter 6: Nouns and Pronouns

EXERCISE 5 ▶ p. 160.

1. hat
2. toys
3. pages
4. bridge
5. keys
6. dish

EXERCISE 7 ▶ p. 161.

1. prizes   ways
2. lips   pants
3. glasses   matches
4. taxes   shirts
5. plates   stars
6. toes   fingers
7. laws   maps
8. lights   places

EXERCISE 9 ▶ p, p. 161.

1. This shirt comes in three sizes: small, medium, and large.
2. How much will the sales tax be?
3. Taxes are low here.
4. I'm not going to buy this car. The price is too high.
5. I can't find my glasses anywhere. Have you seen them?
6. The prize for the contest is a new bike.

EXERCISE 27 ▶ p. 171.

How Some Animals Stay Cool

How do animals stay cool in hot weather? Many animals don't sweat like humans, so they have other ways to cool themselves.

Dogs, for example, have a lot of fur and can become very hot. They stay cool mainly by panting. If you don't know what *panting* means, this is the sound of panting.

Cats lick their paws and chests. When their fur is wet, they become cooler.

Elephants have very large ears. When they are hot, they can flap their huge ears. The flapping ear acts like a fan, and it cools them. Elephants also like to roll in the mud to stay cool.

EXERCISE 35 ▶ p. 174.

A: I'm looking for a new place to live.
B: How come?
A: My two roommates are moving out. I can't afford my apartment. I need a one-bedroom.
B: I just helped a friend find one. I can help you. What else do you want?
A: I want to be near the subway ... within walking distance. But I want a quiet location. I don't want to be on a busy street.
B: Anything else?
A: A small balcony would be nice.
B: That's expensive.
A: Yeah. I guess I'm dreaming.

EXERCISE 47 ▶ p. 181.

1. Who's knocking on the door?
2. Whose coat is on the floor?
3. Whose glasses are those?
4. Who's sitting next to you?
5. Whose seat is next to yours?
6. Who's outside?

Chapter 7: Modal Auxiliaries, the Imperative, Making Suggestions, Stating Preferences

EXERCISE 3 ▶ p. 194.

A: Where do you and Joe have to go tomorrow?
B: I have to go downtown. Joe has to take the kids to buy school supplies. He couldn't do it today.
A: May I come with you?
B: You can if you want to get up early.
A: Would you wake me up? Sometimes I'm not able to hear my alarm.
B: Sure. I have a great way to wake people up. You definitely won't sleep in!
A: I can't wait!

EXERCISE 7 ▶ p. 197.

In the Classroom

A: I can't understand this math assignment.
B: I can help you with that.
A: Really? Can you explain this problem to me?
B: Well, we can't figure out the answer until we do this part.
A: OK. But it's so hard.
B: Yeah, but I know you can do it. Just go slowly.

A: I need to leave in a few minutes. Can you meet me after school today to finish this?

B: Well, I can't meet you right after school, but how about at 5:00?

A: Great!

EXERCISE 13 ▶ p. 199.

1. A: Mom, are these oranges sweet?
   B: I don't know. I can't tell if an orange is sweet just by looking at it.

2. A: What are you going to order?
   B: I'm not sure. I might have pasta, or I might have pizza.

3. A: Mom, can I have some candy?
   B: No, but you can have an apple.

4. A: What are you doing this weekend?
   B: I don't know yet. I may go snowboarding with friends, or I may try to fix my motorcycle.

5. May I have everyone's attention? The test is about to begin. If you need to leave the room during the examination, please raise your hand. You may not leave the room without asking. Are there any questions? No? Then you may open your test booklets and begin.

EXERCISE 17 ▶ p. 201.

In a Home Office

A: Look at this cord. Do you know what it's for?

B: I don't know. We have so many cables and cords around here with all our electronic equipment. It could be for our old printer.

A: No, that isn't a printer cord.

B: It might be for one of the kids' toys.

A: Yeah, I could ask. But they don't have many electronic toys.

B: I have an idea. It may be for an old cell phone. You know — the one I had before this one.

A: I bet that's it. We can probably throw this out.

B: Well, let's be sure before we do that.

EXERCISE 37 ▶ p. 212.

Filling out a Job Application

1. The application has to be complete. You shouldn't skip any parts. If a section doesn't fit your situation, you can write N/A (not applicable).

2. If you fill out the form by hand, your writing has to be easy to read.

3. You've got to use your full legal name, not your nickname.

4. You've got to list the names and places of your previous employers.

5. You have to list your education, beginning with either high school or college.

6. All spelling has to be correct.

7. A: Do I have to write the same thing twice, like a phone number?
   B: No, you can just write "same as above."

8. A: Do I have to apply in person?
   B: No, for a lot of companies, you can do it online.

EXERCISE 52 ▶ p. 220.

Puzzle steps:

1. Write down the number of the month you were born. For example, write the number 2 if you were born in February. Write 3 if you were born in March, etc.

2. Double the number.

3. Add 5 to it.

4. Multiply it by 50.

5. Add your age.

6. Subtract 250.

Trivia Answers

Chapter 1, Exercise 6, p. 6.

1.	runs	T
2.	run	T
3.	live	F [According to a 1993 study: The death rate for right-handed people = 32.2 percent; for left-handed people = 33.8 percent, so the death rate is about the same.]
4.	cover	T
5.	has	F [The official Eiffel Tower website says 1,665.]
6.	spoils	F [Honey never spoils.]
7.	is	T
8.	takes	T
9.	beats	T
10.	die	T

Chapter 5, Exercise 31, p. 138.

1. c
2. d
3. b
4. a
5. e

Chapter 6, Exercise 17, p. 165.

(*Some items have more than one answer.*)
1. Georgia, Azerbaijan, Kazakhstan, China, Mongolia
2. Denmark
3. The Thames
4. The Dominican Republic, Cuba, Jamaica
5. Laos, Thailand, Cambodia, China
6. (*Answers will vary.*)
7. Liechtenstein
8. Vatican City
9. (*Answers will vary.*)
10. Egypt, Sudan, Eritrea, Iran

Chapter 6, Exercise 42, p. 178.

1.	earth's	T
2.	elephant's	F [gray and wrinkled]
3.	man's	T
4.	woman's	T
5.	women's	T
6.	person's	T
7.	People's	F [Men's voices have a higher pitch.]

Index

After, 57, 80, 116 (*Look on page 57 and also on pages 80 and 116.*)	The numbers following the words listed in the index refer to page numbers in the text.
Consonants, defined, 11*fn.* (*Look at the footnote on page 11.*)	The letters *fn.* mean "footnote." Footnotes are at the bottom of a chart or the bottom of a page.

Credits

Katarzyna Białasiewicz/123RF; **128:** Iakov Kalinin/123RF; **130:** Asier Romero/Shutterstock; **131:** Albertus engbers/123RF; **132:** Foodandmore/123RF; **135:** Pearlphoto/123RF; **136:** Vadim Petrakov/Shutterstock; **137:** Shutterstock; **138:** Johan2011/123RF; **139:** Olegdudko/123RF; **143:** Ruth Black/123RF; **144:** Matej Kastelic/ Shutterstock; **147:** Arena Creative/Shutterstock; **151:** Kamil Macniak/Shutterstock; **152:** Justmeyo/123RF; **153:** Olga Dogadina/Shutterstock; **157:** Elvira Koneva/123RF; **158:** Ymgerman/123RF; **159** (businesspeople): Mark Bowden/123RF; **159** (Mexican food): Tonobalaguer/123RF; **159** (butterfly): Tobkatrina/123RF; **159** (boy & dinosaur skeleton): Pavel L Photo and Video/Shutterstock; **162:** Jaysi/123RF; **163:** Vanessa van Rensburg/Shutterstock; **164:** Freeograph/123RF; **165:** Elenathewise/123RF; **166:** Dracozlat/123RF; **167** (student in library): My Visuals/123RF; **167** (sad birthday): Dmitriy Shironosov/123RF; **167** (fashion designer): Elnur/Shutterstock; **169:** Volodymyr Burdiak/Shutterstock; **170:** Angela Waye/Shutterstock; **171:** Five-Birds Photography/Shutterstock; **173** (roast chicken): Magone/123RF; **173** (brick wall): Sedat seven/123RF; **174:** Vicspacewalker/Shutterstock; **176** (carrot cake): Brent Hofacker/123RF; **176** (chocolate tart): Alexey Astakhov/123RF; **176** (ice cream sandwiches): Natasha Breen/123RF; **176** (bees): Diyana Dimitrova/Shutterstock; **176** (ping pong table): Mark Vorobev/123RF; **177** (left): Ammentorp/123RF; **177** (right): Ammentorp/123RF; **179** (top): Eobrazy/123RF; **179** (bottom right): Shutterstock; **180** (woman and handbag): Akz/123RF; **180** (boy with apple): Parinya Binsuk/123RF; **180** (man getting into car): Andrey_ Popov/Shutterstock; **180** (dog): Jaromir Chalabala/123RF; **180** (ski vacation): ProStockStudio/Shutterstock; **182:** Gresei/Shutterstock; **183** (man and mirror): Dean Drobot/Shutterstock; **183** (woman and mirror): Katielittle/Shutterstock; **183** (cat and mirror): Rasulov/Shutterstock; **184:** Marina Lvova/123RF; **184:** Marina Lvova/123RF; **184:** Marina Lvova/123RF; **185** (washer & drier): Golf Money/Shutterstock; **185** (washer & drier): Golf Money/Shutterstock; **185** (stove): Neamov/Shutterstock; **185** (stove): Neamov/Shutterstock; **186** (microwave): Oleksandr_Delyk/Shutterstock; **186** (dishwasher): Moreno Soppelsa/Shutterstock; **186** (refrigerator): Ppart/Shutterstock; **186** (saw): Phrej/Shutterstock; **186** (hammer): Revers/Shutterstock; **186** (screwdriver): Gareth Boden/Pearson Education Ltd; **186** (wrench): Lotus_studio/Shutterstock; **186** (tulips left): Allegro7/123RF; **186** (tulips right): Liligraphie/123RF; **189:** Dolgachov/123RF; **191** (man): Blaj Gabriel/Shutterstock; **191** (woman): Maridav/123RF; **193:** Germanskydiver/Shutterstock; **195:** 2xSamara. com/Shutterstock; **196** (chess): Vetkit/Shutterstock; **196** (guitar player): Arieliona/Shutterstock; **198:** Kichigin/ Shutterstock; **199:** Sirtravelalot/Shutterstock; **200:** Dotshock/Shutterstock; **201:** Nadezda Ledyaeva/123RF; **202:** Eunika/123RF; **204:** Shutterstock; **207:** Image Point Fr/Shutterstock; **209:** Woodoo007/123RF; **213:** Stokkete/ Shutterstock; **215:** Golubovy/123RF; **217:** Dolgachov/123RF; **219:** Belchonock/123RF; **220:** Dieter Hawlan/ Shutterstock; **222:** Africa Studio/Shutterstock; **225:** StockLite/Shutterstock.

Illustration credits: Aptara, page **188**; Don Martinetti—**70, 140, 187**; Chris Pavely—**33, 43**